"Vivid and emotionally spot-on. *Baby Bomb* doesn't miss a beat in giving you helpful tools, examples, and dialogue right from the first chapter. This book tackles the pervasive problem of traditional gender roles in parenting, elevates the conversation, and challenges us to think deeper about nurturing our partner relationships after baby comes along."

—**Heather Turgeon**, psychotherapist, and author of
The Happy Sleeper

"'*The couple comes first.*' Strange how radical these words seem, but also how right. *Baby Bomb* insists—and gives parents concrete ways to remember—that their health and partnership is never any less important than their baby. This book is a breath of fresh air that helps lighten even the hardest days of early parenting."

—**Angela Garbes**, author of *Like a Mother*

"After the birth of a baby, the relationship of the parents is often left untended, like a fallow field. *Baby Bomb* is the guide you need to help return nutrients to the soil of your relationship, plant seeds of new growth, and celebrate the bounty of your relationship for years to come."

—**Britta Bushnell, PhD**, childbirth and new-parent specialist,
and author of *Transformed by Birth*

"Buy this book now. Give *Baby Bomb* to every expectant couple you know. It is an indispensable guide for all new parents and pregnant couples. There is none other like it. It will nourish the couple; teach them how to care for one another, make collaborative decisions, and flourish as a strong team."

—**Ellyn Bader, PhD**, cofounder The Couples Institute,
creator of the Developmental Model of Couples Therapy,
and coauthor of *Tell Me No Lies*

"*Baby Bomb* is a gift for young couples. The principles of attachment theory and nervous system regulation are the basic elements of 'Parenting 101.' And Kara's fresh voice of experience explaining how to apply those principles is the bow on top."

> —**Diane Poole Heller, PhD**, creator of the Dynamic Attachment Re-Patterning experience (DARe), president of Trauma Solutions, and author of *Healing Your Attachment Wounds* and *The Power of Attachment*

"The inevitable clash of competing loyalties that come with being a partner, a parent, and yourself can be painful when they're out of balance. With exceptionally incisive insight, Kara and Stan help you map confusing emotional experiences. For thirty-five years, I worked as a psychologist supporting and helping couples through their toughest times. I wish I had this book all along. I'm glad I have it now."

> —**Peter Pearson, PhD**, cofounder The Couples Institute, and coauthor of *Tell Me No Lies*

"I was moved by the powerful insights in this book, which teaches couples how to integrate partnership and parenting. Kara and Stan shift the old paradigm—whereby mothers are the ones primarily responsible for raising a securely attached child—to a new paradigm in which secure-functioning couples do that together, and do so more effectively. Partnering according to these principles gives birth to a vast transformation through which both partners and their child grow. I encourage therapists and doctors to get more than one copy of this book to share with every couple who is expecting."

> —**Nilufer Devecigil**, therapist, and author of *Işığın Yolu*

"There is a saying that the best thing you can do for your children is to have a great relationship with each other. *Baby Bomb* is a manual for making that happen. Every parent-to-be should read it, and everyone who is already a parent should read it. Your children will thrive, if you do."

> —**Harville Hendrix, PhD**, and **Helen LaKelly Hunt, PhD**, coauthors of *Giving the Love That Heals*

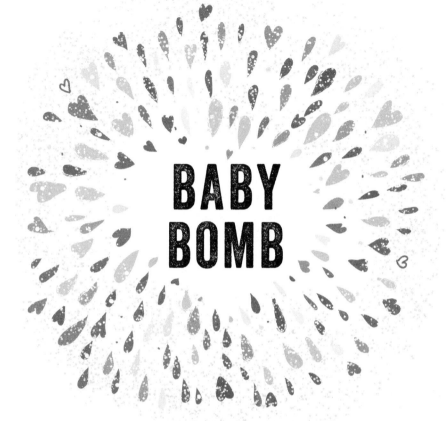

BABY BOMB

A RELATIONSHIP SURVIVAL GUIDE for NEW PARENTS

Kara Hoppe, MFT | Stan Tatkin, PsyD

New Harbinger Publications, Inc.

Publisher's Note

NEW HARBINGER PUBLICATIONS is a
registered trademark of New Harbinger Publications, Inc.

Distributed in Canada by Raincoast Books

Copyright © 2021 by Kara Hoppe and Stan Tatkin
New Harbinger Publications, Inc.
5674 Shattuck Avenue
Oakland, CA 94609
www.newharbinger.com

Cover design by Amy Shoup

Acquired by Jennye Garibaldi

Edited by Jennifer Eastman

Library of Congress Cataloging-in-Publication Data

Names: Hoppe, Kara, author. | Tatkin, Stan, author.
Title: Baby bomb : a relationship survival guide for new parents / Kara Hoppe and Stan Tatkin.
Description: Oakland, CA : New Harbinger Publications, [2021] | Includes bibliographical references.
Identifiers: LCCN 2020055602 | ISBN 9781684037315 (trade paperback)
Subjects: LCSH: Parenthood. | Couples. | Interpersonal relations. | Parenting.
Classification: LCC HQ755.8 .H659 2021 | DDC 306.874--dc23
LC record available at https://lccn.loc.gov/2020055602

Printed in the United States of America

24   23   22

10   9   8   7   6   5   4   3   2

To Charlie and Jude—you two are my everything. I can't imagine loving you more.

—K. H.

To my mother and father, who showed me what it meant to be in love, be devoted, be dependable, and do the right thing. To my wife, Tracey, and my stepdaughter, Joanna, who continue to show me how to be secure functioning and live a blessed life.

—S. T.

Contents

Foreword

For couple therapists, it's an open secret: children can eviscerate a relationship. Sex researcher Barry McCarthy is fond of torturing audiences by telling parents, "The research is clear. Sexual satisfaction plummets with the birth of the first child and springs back as soon as the youngest leaves for college."

Until you've personally crossed that threshold and had your heart melted by that scrunched little face—only to wake at two in the morning to the sound of screaming and the prospect of falling out of bed and stumbling through the dark yet again—you just don't know. As blind urgency pushes you through the haze of sleep deprivation—suddenly mixed with a particularly robust hatred toward your resting partner—you poke them in the ribs and cry, "It's your turn. Get up! I mean it; it's your damn turn!"

There really is no way to fully prepare for a baby, no matter how many books you read. One parent in my clinical practice put it this way: "It's like political torture in some dictatorship. You have this ear-splitting thing that explodes in your face at all hours, without warning. And none of the inane, rather humiliating things you did last time—jostle, coo, stand on one leg—turns off the shrieking. In fact, nothing seems to work."

Welcome to the baby bomb! Whatever you previously thought, throw most of it out the window.

Before the first of our two boys was born, I asked friends for novels I might enjoy during my month of paternity leave. I'd have a few minutes here and there to escape, right? My best friend gave me a book of one-minute short stories, with a note that read simply "Good luck!"

What you most likely won't hear admitted to in playgroups or at the swings in the park is the one word I associate with this moment in the life cycle of any family: *overwhelm*. I'm talking about the sense that it's all too much—that the noise, the endless need for patience, the tensions with your partner are more than you can bear.

The truth is that, like any intense love relationship, the parent-child relationship can serve as an emotional vacuum cleaner, pulling out of you the fissures and unhealed issues from your own childhood. Were your parents neglectful? Odds are you'll be a super-attentive parent. Was your childhood tightly controlled? Odds are you'll be a permissive parent. Which is not to say your partner will be the same. Often quite the opposite occurs. Your sensitivity reads to your partner as coddling. Their discipline feels to you like cruelty. Your sacred agenda for your little one—that they won't experience the parental mistakes you did—is at odds with your partner's agenda. It can lead to what I call *parental hell,* when you witness your partner actively doing to your child some version of the terrible things you experienced at that age—the very things you swore your child would never be subjected to. And you want to murder your partner.

Relax. All this is normal. It comes with the territory. You can and will master this; you can and will even thrive, not just as a family but also as a couple. But you have to know how. That's where *Baby Bomb* comes in. It will reach you in the most confused, harried parts of your soul. Because it has the palliative for overwhelm. It's called wisdom.

This book consists of ten fundamental principles that represent a lifetime of work by Stan—a lifeline that has been brought to life by Kara. Learn how to operationalize these principles. Together, they make an invaluable guide to the heart-swelling, maddening, challenging domain of parenting. These principles are so well informed by neurobiology and so superior to the defaults you absorbed growing up and navigating our mainstream culture that doing them even imperfectly can transform your life. And you can start doing them imperfectly today. Just remember: you needn't face all this on your own. With this book, you're blessedly bombed. You and your partner will gain the insight and practical tools of a united bomb squad, ready to face any explosions or overwhelm life throws your family's way.

—Terry Real, LICSW

Family therapist, speaker, and author of
*The New Rules of Marriage: What You Need
to Know to Make Love Work*

Introduction

When my son was a year old, I was interviewed by the host of a podcast who asked me what tarot cards I would use to describe my experience of motherhood. Without hesitation I said, "the Fool, Death, and the Tower." Even if you have never heard of tarot cards, you can probably gather from those words that my experience of motherhood has been profound. The Fool spoke to my open-hearted call to adventure and the naiveté I felt about motherhood before becoming a mother. The Death card wove in the instant ending and beginning that came with my son's birth. And the Tower represented the crashing down and dismantling of all structures, which for me was my journey of early motherhood. Becoming a parent has been a tapestry of joy, grief, worry, love, confusion, fear, and more love. It has left me both awestruck and humbled. It has also been empowering, boring, lonely, connective, surprising, and infinitely more. In other words, the adventure has been a full-tilt boogie.

The day my husband, Charlie, and I brought our son home, I was still full-on Fool card. I didn't know what to expect of parenthood or how it would change my partnership with Charlie. And nor did he. Eager as we were to embark on this journey, neither of us realized the extent to which both our individual identities and our marriage were about to be overhauled. It didn't take long for the Tower card experience to begin: the dismantling effect of parenthood touched nearly every part of our marriage—from sex to conflict and everything in between.

When Jude was only a few days old, Charlie and I were sitting all cozy on our couch on a winter afternoon, as we'd done many times before—me on my side, Charlie on his. Only now there was a third person, and his place was on *me* to nurse. Nursing didn't come easily for Jude and me. It was challenging to learn how to direct his lips to my breast so he could get a good latch. I had to listen for the sound of him swallowing and watch for his little jaw moving, signs that he was nourishing himself. If I didn't hear swallowing or see his jaw move, it was time to pull him off gently and retry for a better latch. Eventually I came to think of breastfeeding as one latch at a time, and I did that until we became nursing pros. But on this winter day, pros we were not, and nursing was frustrating. Try as I might, I couldn't get a good latch.

Finally we managed it. I relaxed as I heard Jude's swallowing and felt pride and joy. I could do this! As I glanced over at Charlie—blissed out as I was from oxytocin and my sense of accomplishment—I suddenly realized how thirsty nursing made me. And I also realized I couldn't fix that myself: Jude was firmly planted on me, and I was firmly planted on the couch.

"Hey babe," I said, "could you get me a glass of water?"

It was such a simple request. Yet it hit me like a proverbial bomb. I needed Charlie—and needed him in ways I hadn't needed anyone before. When Charlie returned with that glass of water, I looked at him, tears streaming down my face and my throat tight with emotion. All I could say was "I love you so much." My throat wouldn't allow any other words to get out.

I felt a dizzying vulnerability. All the ways I needed Charlie flashed before my eyes. I needed him to help me parent. I needed him to help me take care of myself. I needed him to go through this new adventure of parenting with me, like nothing we'd ever shared before. We were bonded together forever by being Jude's parents.

Elizabeth Stone, a professor at Fordham University, was famously quoted by journalist Ellen Cantarow as saying, "Making the decision to have a child— it's momentous. It is to decide forever to have your heart go walking around outside your body." Charlie and I both now have parts of our hearts walking outside our bodies, and we need to support each other in new and more complex ways. Life will never be as simple as it was before. We both experienced the Death card in the sudden ending of our two-person coupledom, followed by the beginning of our family of three.

Baby Bomb is the book Charlie and I could have used when we became parents. Even though we had enjoyed a more-happy-than-not marriage pre-parenthood, we found ourselves struggling after we became parents. We were fortunate to be able to turn for guidance to the principles and practices I knew as a couple therapist. In particular, we leaned hard on the concept of a *secure-functioning relationship*, which was developed by my mentor Stan Tatkin as part of his psychobiological method for working with couples. In a nutshell, a secure-functioning relationship is one in which the partners are wholeheartedly committed to caring for themselves and each other as their top priority. As we know from research on attachment theory (i.e., that the same strength of bonding that is important between a parent and child in the early years is also important between two adults in an intimate relationship) as well as from neuroscientific evidence, this kind of secure functioning is a couple's best bet for success. I'll talk more in the following chapters about what attachment theory and neuroscience have to offer as you welcome your baby bomb into your party of two.

Charlie and I had made a commitment to practice secure functioning on a day-to-day basis pre-Jude. We each advocated for our own needs and wants, and we took each other's needs and wants equally seriously. We respected our agreement to care for one another first and foremost. However, when we became parents, we found we had to double down on all that. It suddenly became more difficult to practice secure functioning. The pull to put baby first was so strong that we almost drifted apart and lost our coupledom when Jude hit the scene. He was the sun around which we orbited. Our living room became all-things-baby, complete with a diaper dispenser and changing table. My body was focused entirely on Jude: I ate to nurse, and I slept only to wake and nurture him. I was consumed with tending to his well-being. This seemed to make sense at the time, but it wasn't sustainable, because it undermined the secure functioning Charlie and I had committed to. Rather than caring for each other first and foremost, we turned away from each other and made Jude our top priority. If anything, our need for care from each other became greater after Jude was born, but neither of us respected that responsibility as we had done pre-parenthood. The result was that Charlie and I both felt neglected and hurt. We were stuck in our own silos, isolated new parents bickering with each other as we just tried to make it through another day.

It took a lot of effort and hard work in the months that followed to protect our coupledom so all three of us could win in the end. We looked for guidance from our mentor couples, friends, and fellow parents, as well as from a variety of books, and we slowly clawed our way back to each other as transformed (and continually transforming) but still madly in love partners. Our marriage is deeper in terms of trust, love, respect, and intimacy now that we are parents. However, all that tenderness and wonderfulness didn't magically arrive with the baby. Charlie and I had to grow as a team and as lovers.

New parents have always sought advice about parenting. It's one of the most challenging gigs in life, yet no formal preparation exists for the job. William Sears, coauthor of the 1990s classic *The Baby Book*, says the most-asked questions he hears from new parents include whether baby is getting enough breastmilk, how to know if bonding is occurring, how to get baby to sleep through the night, and when it's okay to pick baby up. These are relevant concerns for any new parent. But what I find glaringly missing from most parenting advice is how to partner so you increase your chances of both successful parenting and successful partnering. In fact, *Baby Bomb* is based on the premise that successful partnering is not merely an important part of the equation—it is the first step for couples who want to be successful parents.

This is not to say you can't be a great single parent or that struggling with your partner dooms you to be a bad parent. You can, and it doesn't. However, coupledom is a significant part of most parents' lives, and unease or distress within that primary relationship can create a ripple effect of struggle that extends into all areas of your lives, including parenting. I have noticed that when Charlie and I are at odds with one another, it is more difficult to be a parent. For example, my patience can wear thin, and I can take average toddler misbehavior personally instead of seeing it as developmentally appropriate—something I'm less likely to do when Charlie and I are solid. Becoming a parent can be a wild and epic transformation (think an entire Tarot deck of experiences), so you and your partner want to be on as solid ground as possible. You both need all the support you can get for yourselves and each other.

In this introduction, I first look at the impact a firstborn has on the couple's life. I then introduce the concept of secure functioning and the ten guiding principles for effective partnering and parenting. I look at how you can use these principles to integrate becoming a parent into your partnership. Finally, I offer some suggestions for how to use this book.

Your Baby's Impact

The moment when I was nursing and asked Charlie for water—and many other moments like it—showed me that bringing home a baby is a wonderful and profound experience that no one is 100 percent ready or prepared for. There are no test runs. There are no aunt or uncle experiences that equate. And once it happens, there is no going back. When you as a couple decide to have a baby, you are inviting what I've come to call a *baby bomb* into your lives. I don't use that phrase lightly. Yes, a bomb can have negative connotations (e.g., "it bombed," meaning it was a total fail), but it is increasingly used with positive connotations ("it's the bomb," meaning it's the best). In essence, it refers to something earthshattering, momentous, and with huge impact, and I like how it captures the multidimensional impact of a new baby. My heart was blown wide open as I fell more and more in love with Jude every day; at the same time, my life pre-Jude was blown to shreds, with the debris landing everywhere. With my life revolving around Jude, my relationships with friends and family were fragmented, leaving me with a weakened support team. My most basic needs were at the mercy of Jude. One day, I asked Charlie to watch him so I could use the restroom. As I sat in there, I thought, *I can't even take care of my need to pee without a freaking committee meeting. How did this happen?* I missed my old life and felt grief for it. That grief was just as real as my undying love for Jude.

Researchers have repeatedly found that marital satisfaction declines after a baby is born. This is especially true for mothers. One early study, conducted in the 1950s by E. E. LeMasters, found 83 percent of new parents were in what he termed a "moderate to severe crisis." More recently, internationally renowned couple therapist John Gottman and his colleagues reported that 67 percent of couples saw their level of satisfaction "plummet" after the birth of their first child. Think the Tower card. Gottman and other researchers speak about satisfaction as depending on effective couple communication, quality time spent together, and the presence of external support. Perhaps you are experiencing the loss of some of these important elements. For example, it may be harder to find time to talk with your partner, let alone carve out the quality time you used to enjoy. You may find yourself making decisions alone, because you don't want to wait until your partner is around and because your friends are even less available. You may be struggling with the increased responsibility of parenthood—emotionally, financially, and logistically. One of you has to be caring for baby at any given moment, and that requires constant negotiation between you. Really, it's not a surprise to see new parents at each other's throats as a result of all the pressure and instant change their baby bomb delivers.

Still, let's not be too quick to blame the baby bomb. Researchers Philip and Carolyn Cowan conducted a ten-year study of the effects children had on their parents' partnerships and came up with the more nuanced theory that children get "an unfair share of the blame for their parents' distress." They believe "the seeds of new parents' individual and marital problems are sown long before their first baby arrives." Those old unconscious or unresolved issues simply rise to the surface. For example, if you're angry your partner isn't changing enough diapers now, chances are your relationship already had latent issues related to equity. I know from my experience as a therapist that whenever unresolved issues rise to the surface, we have the opportunity to understand and heal them. This view offers hope that you and your partner can weather the transition to parenthood and enjoy a thriving partnership as parents. In this book, I follow the belief that with support and guidance, you can better understand, mitigate, and integrate some of the subtle and not-so-subtle crisis aspects of becoming a parent.

Our pregnancy was planned. Charlie and I had been ride-or-die friends for fifteen years and had shared a home as partners for ten when we got pregnant. We both longed with all our hearts for a child and acknowledged our fears as well. During the pregnancy, we didn't really know what to fear—except for a nebulous giant change on the horizon—so we mostly talked about our hopes. We stayed up late conversing about all the adventures we'd take our son on, while I blissfully rubbed my belly. Charlie is a musician, so he was excited to introduce him to the guitar and piano. Being a therapist, I wanted to cultivate a relationship with our son in which he could feel safe talking about anything. I talked to him during the whole pregnancy, reading stories to him and offering him my insights on life. I felt Charlie and I were acing this whole life-with-baby thing—though in hindsight, we were a bit blind to the fact that he had yet to arrive. The bomb was ticking, but we were so excited to hold Jude that we looked past the reality that parenting goes above and beyond picking out a crib, making a birth plan, and holding a baby.

All those late-night conversations were fantastic fun, but they did little to prepare me for mothering our son or for fostering Charlie's and my partnership once we were parents. Virtually overnight, we became different people with different identities. To make matters worse, we had virtually no time to talk about any of this. We were both too busy being parents and tending to our son. Charlie had always been my go-to person, and that was what I missed most right after Jude was born. I missed long, deep, juicy conversations with my best friend. I missed his support. At that moment, because we were in the thick of it, it was impossible to see the forest for the trees. Most likely, you have (or will soon have) your own trees—areas of your life affected by your baby bomb that make it hard to gain perspective on your new life.

Ultimately, Charlie and I turned to a resource most new parents don't have: my professional training as a couple therapist. Many of the lessons, principles, and tools I had learned were newly relevant to the health and happiness of our marriage. We were able to take what I knew and use it to revamp our marriage to reflect our new status as parents. These lessons and experiences form the backbone of this book.

Before I summarize the ten principles around which this book is organized, I'd like you to think about the impact of a baby on your partnership. If you are an expecting (or hope-to-be-expecting) first-time parent, this will mean looking ahead and imagining. If you are already parents, this will mean looking at your experience with fresh eyes.

DETECTING YOUR BABY BOMB

The following is a list of aspects of your life that are likely to feel (or already have felt) the impact of your baby bomb. Feel free to add to the list. If you think writing about it could help as you sort through the list, maybe start a baby bomb journal that you can turn to as you do the various exercises and work through this book.

If you are an expecting (or hope-to-be) parent, discuss your thoughts about each area of impact with your partner. How relevant does it feel to each of you? How might you deal with it?

If you are already parents, I suggest going through the list with your partner and rating each area on a scale of 1 to 10 (where 1 = little impact and 10 = strong impact). Note that impact can be either positive or negative.

- the birth-mom's body

- your sleep life

- your partner's sleep life

- your moods and emotions

- your partner's moods and emotions

- your exercise routine

- your partner's exercise routine

- your work

- your partner's work

- your creativity and hobbies

- your partner's creativity and hobbies

- your friendships

- your partner's friendships

- your relationship and role in your family

- your partner's relationship and role in their family

- money

- your priorities and responsibilities

- your partner's priorities and responsibilities

- your and your partner's ability to have privacy for sex

The Ten Guiding Principles

Many couples expect their baby to bring them closer, but without the guidance and tools to deal with the massive transformation they are experiencing, they drift apart instead. To avoid this, you need guidance to navigate and integrate these changes.

As I was processing how my skills as a couple therapist could help Charlie and me in our transition to parenthood, I consulted Stan. I wanted to understand how his psychobiological approach might apply not just to adult intimate relationships but also, more specifically, to new parents. As we talked, and as I thought about it, I realized that the same skill was key in both circumstances: the couple's ability to be *secure functioning*—that is, to be in a relationship grounded in Teamwork with a capital T. I will unpack this more in chapter 1, but the basic idea is that when two partners team up with sensitivity, fairness, justice, and true mutuality, they can thrive, both separately and together. This is exactly what Charlie and I found carried us through the rough spots as new parents and allowed us to reconnect at a new and deeper level.

Stan and I synthesized the following ten guiding principles for successful, secure-functioning partnering and parenting. I'll cover each in more detail, including examples of real couples, in the following chapters. Think of these as your North Star, guiding your relationship, though not in a rigid manner.

1. *The couple comes first.* You and your partner team up to put your relationship first; you treat each other with reciprocity and equality, before all the other aspects of your lives—including before your baby.

All the other guiding principles support this one; it is like the oxygen masks you put on yourselves before you take care of your baby.

2. *You and your partner take care of yourselves and each other.* You monitor yourselves and each other at the level of your nervous systems, and you become experts who know how to soothe or energize each other, as needed.

3. *You and your partner make agreements with each other that you respect.* You communicate openly and directly, including as you formulate and maintain your commitment to each other.

4. *You and your partner make decisions as a team.* You consult with each other on all decisions, including those related to your baby.

5. *You and your partner value your own and each other's needs.* You practice direct communication with each other about your respective needs, and you treat the other's needs as of equal importance to your own.

6. *You and your partner coregulate.* You engage in daily practices that help you manage your nervous systems for relationship restoration as well as preventive care.

7. *You and your partner keep your family and work lives in balance.* You make sure that having a baby does not derail your family-work balance.

8. *You and your partner redefine romance to keep your couple connection alive.* At a time when your sexuality may be at a low ebb, you take time apart from your baby to reconnect and grow your love.

9. *You and your partner fight for two winners.* You always quickly heal any hurt and look for a win-win so neither of you (or your relationship) loses out.

10. *You and your partner parent and partner with sensitivity, respect, and trust.* You strive to create and maintain a secure-functioning relationship, now and throughout your lives together.

Charlie and I are still learning from and revisiting this list. These principles don't provide a one-time fix; they offer practices we can work on, both by ourselves and together. They are the basis of a commitment to good relationship health that we're continually recommitting to. And we both mess up. But that doesn't stop us from helping each other back up to begin practicing again.

Take, for example, our decision to hire a sitter to be on call when Jude was about one year old. I had gone back to work part time when he was four months old, and Charlie had started work before that, but we had alternated our work schedules to avoid hiring childcare. So hiring a sitter was a big move for us.

About a week before our new sitter's first day with Jude, I started to feel irritated and anxious. I found myself wishing Charlie would be a stay-at-home dad or I a stay-at-home mom. I was struck by the irrationality of that wish, because we both love our jobs, and we were spending the majority of our time at home with Jude anyway.

One evening, I snapped at Charlie about something so unimportant I don't even recall what it was. Immediately I apologized. I said, "I'm sorry. I'm being a bitch. But I know what's bothering me. The idea of leaving Jude with a sitter is stressing me out."

He listened and reflected back to me: "I get it. I could see all afternoon that you've been feeling irritable. I was going to suggest we talk about it."

As soon as I felt seen and heard by Charlie, I started to feel less anxious. And when I felt less anxious, we were able to come up with a plan. I said, "Why don't I book the sitter extra early on the first day so I can go over everything thoroughly with her again. That will put me at ease."

Charlie liked that and had another idea: "Let's plan to talk on the phone as you drive to work, so you're not going through the experience alone, and I can reassure you."

On the sitter's first day, we stuck to the plan. As I took her around our house and retold all the details of Jude's life, I felt better. When I shared that leaving was hard for me, I opened myself up to support from her. She offered to send me updates and pictures during the day, and I found myself tearing up in gratitude.

After I kissed Jude goodbye, I cried a bit in the car. Then I called Charlie and told him how it went and how I was doing.

After listening, he reassured me and said, "I think we're doing the right thing. We have a reliable sitter, and we like our jobs, and it's important for Jude to be cared for by other loving caregivers in addition to us."

I felt supported and soothed and closer to Charlie. We benefited from self-reflection, trust, and showing up for each other and ourselves. If we hadn't been able to do that, the morning could have been a shit show (no diaper pun intended). We were working all of the guiding principles at the same time, but the first principle—the couple comes first—supported us in navigating this choppy, emotional experience. Our agreement to put the relationship first let me be vulnerable and share my concerns and feelings with Charlie. His caring and attuned response also put the relationship first. He didn't try to fix my feelings or say anything that negated them; rather, he empathized with me and jumped in to help. Together we cared for each other. When you become more familiar with the guiding principles, you may want to come back to this anecdote and see how the other nine also guided Charlie and me.

Integrating Partnering and Parenting

It doesn't matter if you thoughtfully planned for your baby, like we did, or if you wholeheartedly (or with some ambivalence) embraced a big surprise, there is really no way to truly understand what it will be like until you are parents. Furthermore, there is no way to know how being parents will affect your partnership. Responsibilities are gained, and autonomy is lost. Immense joy and love can abound amid feelings of loss and overwhelm.

How do you go about integrating partnering and parenting? The first step is to recognize that you're bound for change (if you are an expecting couple) or are in the midst of change (if you are already a parent). You understand that the birth of a child can lead to a huge transformation, both for your relationship and for you as new parents.

Second, the best way to turn this transformation into an opportunity for maximum growth is to have lots of support. And that means beginning with your partnership. You and your partner need to be able to support and care for one another before you will be able to do so effectively for your new baby. The key for this is creating a secure-functioning relationship. Stan wrote about secure functioning in *Wired for Love*, his manual for partners who want to become an effective dyad. *Baby Bomb* builds on that work by showing you how to create a secure-functioning relationship that integrates partnering and parenting.

In this book, you will learn how to bring secure functioning into your relationship with your baby. This includes how you let your child know they are safe, important, valuable, and worthy of love and belonging. It includes how you show up for your child when they cry. And how you pick them up when they fall and signal that they need comfort. It includes how you put your child to sleep at night with care and ritual. And how you attune to their needs when they want to share an exciting word or some new skill or trick they've learned. All these little choices you make to lean toward your child and your child's needs and wants are the building blocks of a secure-functioning relationship. This kind of relationship is beneficial for both the couple and the baby. It's a triple win.

How to Use This Book

This book is a journey to finding your way as a couple, as co-creators, as lovers, as friends, and as parents. It is not meant to be a quick fix; it's meant to give you and your partner a set of practices you can bring into your lives, adapting them, as needed, for your unique situation. The book is organized into three sections: "Your Party of Two" helps you form a strong partner team, "Two Become Three" guides you through the transition as baby arrives, and "Thriving in Your Party of Three" explains how to use the guiding principles in an ongoing way within your partnership and family.

Each chapter includes tools, skills, and examples for how you and your partner can welcome the new addition to your family and all the change it brings, as well as learn to grow together. I share many examples of how real-life couples (in addition to Charlie and me) put them into practice, times when they fall out of practice, and how they find their way back to each other and these guiding principles. I know early parenthood is unruly in its demands on your resources, but it's best if you can muster the time and concentration to read the chapters in sequence, because each builds upon the one before.

The book's guiding principles and awareness of cultural differences and cultural messaging make it relevant for a diverse audience. This includes both younger couples who have a child before their careers are intact as well as older couples who already have established careers. My examples are primarily about the arrival of a first child, but the same principles can be applied if you are adding a second child (or more) or if you are expanding your family through adoption or surrogacy. The principles apply to couples who have one partner staying at home with baby and to couples who both work, as well as to both same-sex couples and hetero couples. They also apply if you live in a city or the burbs—or if you are living through a recession, world crisis, or pandemic. So if you are here as an expecting couple or are in the throes of early parenthood, welcome. This book is here to help guide you to integrate your precious baby bomb.

You might wonder how so many apparently different families could find value in the same book. As we'll see in the following chapters, the answer lies in the broad applicability of secure functioning. The principles of secure functioning create an underlying framework upon which you can partner and parent, regardless of the other circumstances of your home life and even the state of the world.

Parenting and partnering is the adventure of a lifetime. I hope you'll find comfort in knowing that you're not alone in your struggle—that partnering and parenting are full of challenges for nearly everyone. Moreover, even if your own parents didn't provide you with an example you wish to emulate, you can find your way through the wild unknown together with your partner. Everyone can learn to do this, even if it wasn't modeled for them. I did.

Finally, this book is not meant to be a replacement for couple therapy, trauma therapy, or other forms of professional support. Parenting and partnering can bring up old traumas or attachment wounding. In case you think this may be happening to you or your partner, I have included resources for professional help in the back of the book.

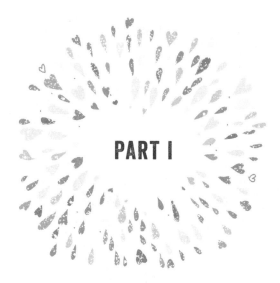

PART I

Your Party
of Two

CHAPTER 1

Your Partner Team

The air is tense in the family room as Lillian brings Leo's pajamas and blankie to him. Oliver sits on the couch, his eyes on his eighteen-month-old son, but not really focused on him. He is lost in thought, trying to process what's going on between him and Lillian and why dinnertime was especially hard tonight. *I said I want to be a more involved parent, yet she blew me off,* he thinks. *It's like she doesn't think I know how to be a good dad.*

"Okay Leo, time to put on your jammies," Lillian says.

"No!" Leo grabs his pajamas and throws them at Oliver.

"It's bedtime," Lillian says, trying to show patience. "Please bring me your PJs."

But Leo digs in. "No, Mama! No!"

Lillian exhales forcefully, then turns to Oliver. "What? Are you just going to watch this from afar?"

Oliver's body jolts, as if awakened from a dream. He looks genuinely startled. Which makes Lillian even more irritated. *Why,* she wonders, *do I let myself get suckered in when he talks about parenting together? He never means it.* She grabs the pajamas and doesn't hide her annoyance: "Guess I'm single parenting tonight, since you're here but not here. I'm amazed you can do your disappearing trick even without your phone."

"What are you taking about? I'm right here. And I'm not *always* on my phone!" Oliver says defensively.

"Whatever." Lillian rolls her eyes. "Why don't I do bedtime alone with Leo, and you go attend to whatever it is you really want to do."

Oliver feels resentment building. "I told you at dinner, Lilly: I want to spend time with you and Leo. It's just hard to take my work hat off when I'm on a deadline and my project isn't going well. I don't know why that's hard for you to understand."

Lillian shoots Oliver a look that signals she could care less, before turning her back on him. She picks Leo up and says, "Say nighty-night to Daddy. I'm going to get you ready for bed."

Oliver walks to his office with a heavy heart and opens the file he was working on earlier. Work feels easier to deal with than trying to partner with Lillian. He hasn't gotten far when she pokes her head in the door. He didn't expect Leo to get to bed so fast, so again he's startled. "Why do you have to sneak up on me?" he says when he sees how annoyed his startled reaction makes her. "You told me to go and work, so that's what I did. And now you're interrupting. Really, I don't know *what* you want."

"I want a resolution to all this tension between us. But I guess I'm the only one who cares. I swear, I don't see the point of being in this relationship!" Without waiting for an answer, Lillian turns and heads back to the living room, where she mulls over all the ways Oliver has let her down and begins to build a bulletproof case against him in her mind.

♥♥♥

Knock-down, drag-out fights like this one between Lillian and Oliver are painful and hard on partners. There was no clear disagreement in this scenario; it was more a case of hurt partners further hurting each other. Instead of tending to their own pain and each other's pain, they either lashed out or shut down. Both styles of response (lashing out and shutting down) are destructive—and even more so as each partner becomes increasingly entrenched in their style.

Inviting another buddy (your baby) into the mix can up not only your level of stress but also the probability of fights like this if you don't recognize that you and your partner are first and foremost a twosome. Many issues encountered by new parents can be traced back to their failure to form a solid twosome before becoming a party of three. Even if you and your partner already created a solid twosome before becoming parents, you still have to learn how to tend to that twosome on a daily basis while caring for baby. And if, like Oliver and Lillian, you're struggling, it's not too late to build a secure-functioning relationship. Whether you're still a party of two or have already become a party of three, I'm going to give you the guiding principles and practical tools you need to transform your partnership into a secure-functioning one.

In this chapter, I discuss the first guiding principle and introduce the first of two theoretical tools that will help you build your secure-functioning relationship: the attachment continuum. The second tool, nervous-system regulation, is introduced in the next chapter. Armed with these two bad boys, you and your partner can better understand yourselves and respond to each other with loving care.

Guiding Principle 1: The couple comes first.

When two people are in the process of falling in love and partnering up, there is usually a period of time—some call it the *honeymoon phase*—when both partners show up for the relationship more often than not. They naturally put their party of two first, because it's the hot new thing in their lives. It feels good during this time to help your partner and to ask for help, to spend time together, and to make each other feel special. Fights like Lillian and Oliver's are rare, if they happen at all.

In every intimate partnership, this phase ends sooner or later and is replaced with reduced excitement and less inspiration. Life tends to feel more ordinary, with the potential for lots of distractions from your party of two. Suddenly you're thinking more about your career and how to get it going or all the ways you can expand it or about a creative endeavor or new hobby or hanging with friends. Or having a baby. You start to prioritize some of these activities over your twosome. Instead of growing into a solid team, your relationship becomes you two … plus an extended number of teammates. Of course, friends and family will always play big roles in your lives, and of course, jobs and other activities will fill hours of your day. This expanded team becomes problematic only when you or your partner no longer put your relationship first, allowing other people (or other interests or activities) to take more of your time and attention than you give to each other.

You can't count on a smooth transition from being a party of two to being a party of three to happen automatically, without effort on your part. For most couples, there is work to do. You both have to learn how to take care of each other while caring for your child. Forming a secure-functioning team like this is the practical expression of our first guiding principle: the couple comes first. You may worry that secure functioning isn't attainable for you, that it's about being a perfect partner or having a perfect partnership. That's not the case! Perfect partners and partnerships don't exist. What does exist and is incredibly valuable is a team that provides both of you with a sense of love and belonging and security. Your team is tended to by both partners, and both partners are equally responsible for its health. All the choices you make as a secure-functioning team boil down to believing in and acting under the assumption that you are in each other's care. On a day-to-day basis, this means:

- You are clear about your own needs and wants, you listen to your partner's needs and wants, and you tend to both as best you can.

- You are aware of your own relationship patterns and your partner's. You use this awareness to foster connection and intuit future disconnection.

- If you feel uncomfortable about something your partner is doing, you take it to them directly.

- You are kind and respectful in your communication. When you fall short—because, let's be honest, you will at times—you make a full and genuine apology.

- You make decisions jointly and seek a win-win solution whenever there is conflict or anything in your lives or relationship falls out of balance.

- You form a united team, and when one of you becomes lax in that commitment, you hold each other accountable in a non-shaming way to the principles of secure functioning you agreed on.

We will unpack each of these qualities—and more—of a secure-functioning team in this chapter and the chapters that follow. Let's start, however, by examining the attachment continuum, the first of our two theoretical underpinnings, and see what it tells us about the importance of putting the couple first.

The Attachment Continuum

When Stan was developing his psychobiological approach to help couples form long-lasting, loving relationships, he drew heavily on the work of attachment theorists, such as John Bowlby and Mary Ainsworth. According to attachment theory, children need a strong and dependable bonding experience with their primary caregivers in order to feel safe in life. When you have this secure base at a young age, you can more easily explore creative play, trust others, be soothed from distress, and develop self-esteem and self-reliance. On the other hand, if you lack a secure base, these aspects of life can be more difficult.

Why should this matter to you? Because the quality of your early attachment bonding can have a lasting effect on how you form relationships as an adult. John Bowlby postulated that attachment is a lifelong process, and other researchers have since confirmed that the degree to which you feel secure plays out in your primary intimate partnership, parenting, and relationships with close friends and coworkers. If you and your partner have a secure base when you become parents, you can more easily relax as you face each new challenge. Putting your coupledom first will occur more naturally, because you don't doubt that your partner has your back. However, if you and your partner don't provide enough of a secure base for each other, putting your coupledom first will likely be difficult. One or both of you may be too preoccupied with trying to nail down a sense of personal security and getting your own needs met first. As a result, your child may grow up feeling a pressure to provide security for you—which, of course, is not a burden you want your child to take on.

In *Wired for Love*, Stan describes three classic attachment styles: secure, ambivalent insecure, and avoidant insecure. (He calls them "anchor," "wave," and "island," respectively). It is important to recognize that these styles aren't fixed. The fact that they developed out of your early childhood bonding experience doesn't predetermine everything. You can be secure in one situation or one relationship and not in another. Or you can be more secure at one time of your life and less at another. And perhaps most important, you can learn and grow in ways that make you more secure, and you and your partner can do this together.

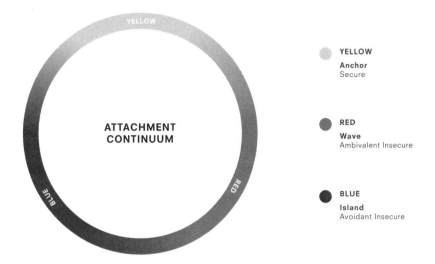

I like to think of the three basic attachment styles as existing on a circular continuum. Because there are no "wrong" or "bad" styles, I like to visualize the continuum with equally vibrant colors. I see secure as shades of yellow, which move toward ambivalent in shades of red, which move toward avoidant in shades of blue, and back again to yellow. These shades allow for an appreciation of the complexity and variations in your attachment style. For example, as you fluctuate between a yellow secure and a blue avoidant style, you might see yourself as green. You can use the descriptions in this chapter for each style to identify where you are now and how you move around on the continuum in response to the ebbs and flows of your relationship and of life.

Although I identify mostly with yellow secure, I can also identify with ambivalent or avoidant, depending on the situation. For example, under the stress of early motherhood, I found myself moving toward a fiery-red ambivalent. One night, I arrived home late from work, exhausted, running on fumes from severe sleep deprivation. I fixed myself a snack and went to get my breast pump for my late-night pumping session. Words can't describe my distress when realized I'd left it at work! In my mind, everything would be okay if Charlie would just drive there and get it. But he didn't offer to do that. Instead, he suggested using a pump we'd gotten from the hospital when Jude was born. I didn't know how to use that pump.

In a sudden burst of frustration born out of fatigue, I chucked the hospital pump to the kitchen floor. Charlie and I can smile about it now, but in that moment, it was a shock for me to see myself spin into red. I was already hovering in orange due to my physical depletion, but feeling unsupported by Charlie pushed me straight into radiant red. Becoming familiar with our attachment styles has helped Charlie and me give and receive support as we make our way around the continuum.

Yellow Secure

Folks on the yellow part of the continuum had primary caregivers who were fairly good at reading their cues and tending to their needs in early childhood. They experienced lots of healthy physical and emotional contact. As adults, they tend to feel comfortable with their body image and secure in their sexuality. They're also confident that they can count on others and that others can count on them. They feel free to acknowledge their need for others and typically find it easy to ask for their needs to be met. They don't have a strong preference for being with others or being alone; they enjoy both options. If they aren't already naturally putting their coupledom first, they are likely to welcome the suggestion, because it reinforces the security and team solidarity they feel with their partner.

Because they feel supported more often than not, yellow peeps can pivot and make appropriate adjustments in the present moment. Commitment to projects, people, and situations comes easily to them. They put a high value on relationships and expect relationships to take work and time to develop. When they encounter rough times, they readily commit to finding resolution. At home or at work, they can assess a problem situation and identify potential win-wins for the involved parties. This is not to say that folks with this attachment style always stay in jobs or in relationships. If staying would not be good for them, they leave. For example, if they find a consistent lack of reciprocity in a relationship, they will leave, because they truly care for themselves and know they deserve better. They are generally self-aware and put that awareness to good use at work and in relationships by taking responsibility for their part in successes and failures.

Am I a Yellow? Is My Partner?

Do any of these traits sound familiar to you? Can you see yourself on this part of the continuum in certain situations? What about your partner? In this exercise, consider these questions:

- Am I equally comfortable in my own company and in the company of others?
- Is it easy for me to commit to relationships, projects, and goals?
- Do I have an easy time adjusting to changing situations and needs?
- Am I comfortable with having needs myself and expressing them, and with others having needs as well?
- Do I find conflict uncomfortable but bearable?

Blue Avoidant

Those on the blue side of the continuum had primary caregivers who were distracted and were physically and emotionally unavailable to care for a child. When blue peeps signaled as youngsters that they needed care, their needs were often ignored. As a result, they stopped signaling and relied instead on themselves to meet their own needs. In adulthood, they avoid situations in which they have to depend too much on others. They are super self-reliant and believe life is best that way. It can be hard for them to collaborate with others since they truly do like to work alone. They can get into a trance-like state when working or creating and are sensitive to being interrupted. Many pursue creative careers that require a lot of alone time for success.

Putting their coupledom first can be threatening to blue folks. They worry that if they have to put the couple first, their own needs won't be met. They also worry that they can't give their partner what that person wants or needs. When blue folks feel they have upset or let down their partner, they tend to distance themselves. This can be physical, such as by leaving the room or home, or it can be in the form of emotional withholding. It can also take the form of quitting the relationship at the first sign of trouble. Blue folks are not natural team players and may outright avoid making commitments, but if they do get involved in a relationship, one of their selling points is being low maintenance. And they are: they don't expect a partner to do for them what they fear they couldn't do for that partner.

Am I a Blue? Is My Partner?

Do any of these traits sound familiar to you? Can you see yourself on this part of the continuum in certain situations? What about your partner? In this exercise, consider these questions:

- Do I think I can take better care of myself than anyone else can?
- Do I have a hard time trusting others for reliable care and nurturing?
- Do I prefer to be alone?
- Do I pride myself on being low maintenance?
- If my partner upsets me, do I need to leave and be alone to recalibrate and come back?

Red Ambivalent

Moving along the continuum, we come to our reds. These folks had primary caregivers who were often in a state of overwhelm and had a hard time attending to their child's needs. As a result, red peeps had their needs met inconsistently, which led them to believe they are burdensome and maybe even unlovable. Their ambivalence stems from the fact that as much as they want loving connection, they fear they won't get it. They adapted by feeling a need to care for others over themselves. In fact, starting at an early age, their primary caregiver may have relied on them to fulfill that caregiver's own emotional needs.

These peeps would love to put their coupledom first, because they deeply want to belong to a secure twosome and be a good team player. However, putting the couple first can be a tricky—even scary—proposition to them. While red folks enjoy caring for others, they struggle to care for themselves. They are afraid they will impose on others, so they have a hard time asking directly for what they need or want, even if that allows their resentment to build. They tend to have a difficult time being alone; they are sensitive to feeling abandoned or forgotten and can become clingy when these fears are stirred up. They can easily become preoccupied with past hurts and injustices, and struggle to be in the present moment or look toward the future. When they get upset, they tend to need to talk it out. They aren't necessarily seeking advice or help, but they need to be heard in order to find themselves again. Sometimes they find themselves angry with their partner or with a friend or family member, but it's hard for them to figure out why.

Am I a Red? Is My Partner?

Do any of these traits sound familiar to you? Can you see yourself on this part of the continuum in certain situations? What about your partner? In this exercise, consider these questions:

- Do I feel more comfortable caring for others than being cared for myself?

- Are separations hard for me?

- Do I sometimes feel angry with my partner but don't know why?

- Do I prefer interacting with others to being alone?

- Am I uncomfortable with my needs, and do I have a hard time asking directly that my needs be met?

Revisiting Lillian and Oliver

Now that you're familiar with the attachment continuum, can you wager a guess as to where Lillian and Oliver might fall? I think it's safe to say Lillian identifies with the red spectrum, while Oliver is sitting pretty in blue.

We can substantiate this by looking at the behaviors and speech of each. Oliver resorts to emotional as well as physical distancing when he feels uncomfortable. He feels safer when he avoids contact and isolates himself in his office and is thrown off balance when Lillian interrupts him. In fact, what might feel like reaching out for contact by someone who's not blue feels to him like an invasion. He tends to get lost in his mind during his interactions with Lillian and has a hard time hearing what she is saying. He filters her words through a lens that is on guard for criticism and shame, which has the effect of raising a threat alarm for him. He is definitely not putting the couple first.

For her part, Lillian wants to put the couple first but doesn't know how to go about it. This creates an ambivalence that is scary for her—she wants to connect with Oliver but fears he won't reciprocate. She is highly sensitive to his being emotionally MIA and his apparent inability to be present as a parent. All of this heightens her fear of abandonment. We don't know about her childhood, but her reaction suggests that one or more of her early caregivers was inconsistently present for her, causing her to expect Oliver to likewise not come through for her. This also would explain why she shows her anger in indirect ways. Take, for example, her anger that Oliver isn't helping with Leo. Instead of directly asking if they can find a solution together, she expresses her anger indirectly by telling him to go off and do his own thing, which is the exact opposite of what she really wants. She seems to have an easier time caring for her son's needs than for her own needs. See if you can notice and name any other behaviors that place Lillian or Oliver on different parts of the attachment continuum.

The ability to place yourself and your partner on the continuum at any given moment is a useful tool. It can be the first step in learning to put your coupledom first if it helps you understand why your attachment style makes it hard for you to do that. Before we examine in the next chapter how you can use nervous-system cues to take this work to the next level, let's see how Lillian and Oliver's interaction might go if they understood how their attachment styles come into play.

This time as Lillian enters the living room with Leo's pajamas and blankie, she sees Oliver on the couch, his eyes on his son but not really focused on him. She hates it when he distances himself. But instead of lashing out, she takes a deep breath. "Okay Leo, hun, we're going to put on your jammies in a minute," she says. Then she turns to Oliver. "I know our conversation earlier didn't go well."

Oliver startles. It disturbs him when Lillian breaks into his thoughts without first asking permission. But in this instance, he's pleasantly surprised she isn't attacking him. "Yeah," he says. "I was just thinking about that."

"You were?"

Oliver nods. Then he gives a little laugh. "I guess I'm being my blue self again. Sorry about that."

Lillian smiles. "Don't be sorry. It's just hard when your blue butts up against my fiery red. And it was starting to blaze at dinner." She looks at Leo, who's tossing his pajamas in the air, and wishes Oliver would jump in and get his son ready for bed—as he often does when things are going well in their little family. But she senses this isn't the moment to bring that up. Instead she says, "I think we should talk more later. Okay?"

"Agreed," Oliver says. It's hard to look at Lillian, because he knows he's disappointing her, but he manages to get the words out: "Would you mind putting Leo to bed by yourself? I'm behind on a deadline, and I can't do both the work thing and also talk later if I hang with you and Leo now."

Lillian wants to object that he should have planned his time better so he wouldn't be abandoning them now. But she realizes that's her red thoughts talking, and Oliver is making an effort to put their twosome first. In fact, he's sounding pretty yellow right now. "Sure!" she says and picks Leo up. "Say nighty-night to Daddy. I'm the lucky one who gets to put you to bed. And Daddy will be the lucky one another night."

♥♥♥

In this scenario, Lillian and Oliver were able to recognize their respective attachment styles and how those styles affect their interactions. This clarity led them to work together more fluidly as a team. Lillian didn't take Oliver's withdrawal personally and lash out. Oliver took responsibility for his blueness and agreed to talk things out later. Neither partner shamed the other for their current color status; instead, they supported each other by acknowledging and accepting that status. By the end, we can feel hopeful they will revisit what's going on in their relationship at a time that works for both and continue to build a solid partner team.

Note that good teamwork doesn't depend on you and your partner having the same attachment style. The key is knowing what your styles are and how they play out in your team. That awareness is attachment theory in action. It gives you both a secure base—to which you always know you can come home.

What Makes This Principle Hard?

Many things can make it difficult to practice putting the couple first. You and your partner may feel as if you're swimming upstream, encountering a powerful current that pulls you to practice otherwise. That current can flow on a personal level, as thoughts that arise from your attachment style, with messages insisting you lean away from partnering. Or that current can flow from our broader culture, which gives messages that value individual effort over teamwork. Let's explore both of these types of messages.

What Your Mind Tells You

"My partner never listens to me. If we're ever gonna get a new car, I'll have to handle it myself." "My partner never helps out unless I ask him to. He's so selfish." "I can never say the right thing. I guess I'm a horrible partner."

Even if you love your partner and find the idea of becoming a strong team appealing, your red or blue colors may sneak up and hijack your mind. Suddenly, your mind is speaking in hyperbole and telling awful stories about your partner or your partnership. Despite your best intentions, you jump out of team mode and into self-protective mode.

What can you do about this? Working with your own mind is a lifelong project, and learning about your attachment style is just one step. Here are some tips as you begin to negotiate this process.

- When your red or blue colors flare forth, chances are there's a message in there from your childhood or a prior relationship. If you notice a self-protective thought (e.g., thinking you have to do things alone or you can't do anything right), challenge yourself to explore the origin of that message so you can begin to reverse it if it isn't productive for your partner team.

- Notice when you hear your mind speaking in terms of *always* or *never*. Rarely do people always or never do anything. Challenge yourself to think of exceptions to those always or never statements.

- Be open to the possibility that you're hurting in some way. Investigate what may have happened that sparked your hurt. Talk to your partner about it. For example, "My mind is telling me a crazy story that you don't love me anymore" or "I realize it hurt my feelings when you shut down my idea."

What Culture Tells You

Some of the thoughts that trip you up don't come as much from your early childhood or past relationships as from the culture. When I say *culture*, I'm referring to mainstream American popular culture. A lot of subtle and not-so-subtle popular cultural messaging tells us to see ourselves as individuals and not as part of a team. It also tells parents to put baby first, not the couple.

Let's take a look at two such messages and how you can counteract them to strengthen your team. You'll notice that cultural obstacles are a theme throughout the book. In many future chapters, we will look at cultural messages relevant to the guiding principles discussed in those chapters.

It's either-or. "I can't change jobs, because I have to put my partner through grad school." "We always go to my in-laws for vacation." "I need to book a ten-day retreat so I can get some peace and quiet from my family."

This cultural message forces us to make an either-or choice. You have to either put yourself first or put your partner first. Moreover, taking care of yourself is the implied priority, and if you take care of your partner first, you will necessarily lose out. In other words, you can't count on anyone to care for you. Which is simply untrue. This is a false dichotomy that stems from an individualistically oriented culture. In fact, you and your partner can learn to care for each other equally. You don't have to choose between yourselves. You can choose both by putting your coupledom first.

What can you do about this? In fact, you don't have to let this message dictate what happens in your relationship. Here are some tips to identify and fix any ways it is not conducive to your partner team.

- Notice this message popping up in articles, films, television shows, and other media.

- Notice it in your own relationship.

- Share your observations with your partner.

- Discuss with your partner how this messaging appears in your partnership and find win-win solutions you two can choose that benefit both of you.

Baby comes first. "When are you going to settle down?" "Those ovaries don't work forever. Clock is a-ticking." "Babies save marriages."

Every woman I know has had to contend with the cultural message that having a baby is integral to her individuality, that it will make her complete as an individual. Even before we bled and could physically have babies, it was a cultural given that we would someday. Duh. And if we didn't want to be mothers, that was odd at best and selfish at worst. The culture puts so much pressure on women to start a family that when we do become pregnant, it's hard to practice putting the couple first. It's hard to tune out the loud and persistent chorus saying, "Baby, Baby, Baby, Baby! Everything for baby!"

What can you do about this? There are ways to counter this messaging. Together with your partner, become more aware of this cultural message in your lives. You can do this playfully, as a game, keeping track of what you notice and discussing it with each other.

- Identify cultural messages that put baby first in advertisements, television shows and movies, and social media.

- Pay attention to how much each of you is asked about your love life, compared with your career or other interests.

- Observe what makes you feel complete—not just as individuals but also as a team.

Conclusion

When you decide to put your relationship first, you accept yourself and your partner as you both are, not as you wish each other would be. A useful tool to begin this journey of acceptance is the attachment continuum. Knowing what color(s) you are currently, mostly, under stress, while learning, and so on offers insight and understanding. It also helps you form a secure-functioning team, which gives you a solid base from which to become the best parents you can be. Being a secure partner team is a practice that can be learned, even if it wasn't modeled for you during your early years. In the next chapter, you will expand your work as a partner team to become experts who know how to care for yourselves and each other, further strengthening your party of two so that it is fully ready to become a party of three.

CHAPTER 2

Becoming Experts
on Each Other

As we saw in chapter 1, once you and your partner understand the value of becoming a secure-functioning team, it can be helpful to know where you each fall on the attachment continuum. But here's a tough question: how much can you *really* do with that information?

For example, knowing my style and Charlie's style helped us to diffuse a tense situation when I jumped into fiery red, throwing that breast pump to the kitchen floor. Knowing about our styles—that under stress, I'm prone to feeling abandoned, and that Charlie can distance himself when he feels like he's disappointing me—also gave us a basis for future discussions. But that night, helpful as it was, this information wasn't enough. The support I needed—that both of us needed, actually—was more than could be expressed through words. At the micro level of our nervous systems, our bodies needed to be soothed and calmed and reassured.

In fact, if you're serious about building a secure partner team, the advantages of knowing your respective attachment styles are limited. You and your partner also need to be able to help each other in real time, moment to moment. You need to be able to do this as the fears and insecurities from your colors loom large and in charge. The good news is that this is possible. You both can learn how to do it!

Here is where the other theoretical tool that Stan uses as a basis for his psychobiological approach—neuroscience and, more specifically, nervous-system regulation—takes center stage. If the attachment continuum is the compass you can use to figure out where you are in the forest of your partnership, then nervous-system regulation is the tool you can use to feed and water, prune and trim, each and every tree. While your primary attachment style remains relatively consistent over time, even if it varies under certain circumstances, your nervous system changes minute by minute, if not millisecond by millisecond.

When I first learned from Stan about how nervous-system regulation can be helpful for couples, he used a computer-generated picture of two stick figures, side by side, each composed entirely of a vast network of nerves. No bones or skin; just nerves. It was a nerdy image, but the point was clear: we humans relate to each other through our nervous systems. You and your partner are, in essence, two nervous systems interacting. That might sound funny, but it also gives rise to a tool I think you'll find useful.

In this chapter, as we move from a macro level to a micro level, I discuss how you and your partner can take care of yourselves and each other using an awareness of your nervous systems. I show you how to become experts on each other who can step up and help manage—that is, *coregulate*—one another's nervous systems on a daily basis and especially in moments of need. The ability to do this is critical for secure-functioning teamwork and can be a powerful relationship game changer.

Guiding Principle 2: You and your partner take care of yourselves and each other.

Perhaps the most remarkable thing about the nervous system—especially when you consider how vital it is to our interactions—is how little attention we tend to pay to it. You might take stock of how you feel—how happy or sad or mad you are—but do you take stock of the state of your nervous system? In fact, the primary way you experience your emotions is through your nervous system. When you're happy, for example, your nervous system might have a pleasant balance of tranquil and excited energy. When you're angry at your partner, your nervous system is likely to be highly excited. However, it will also be highly excited when you are sexually aroused or when you see your partner after a week-long business trip. Similarly, your nervous system will be low energy when you are sad or depressed, as well as when you are cozy in bed and about to drop off to sleep. In short, although you experience emotions through your nervous system, there isn't a one-on-one correspondence between what you feel and the state of your nervous system. The nervous system is putting out data every second of every day, but those data are only as valuable as your ability to recognize and use them.

The nervous system is more intricate than we can—or need to—discuss here. For the purpose of learning to work with your partner, it is helpful to consider the functioning of the nervous system on a continuum. In this case, instead of a circular continuum, picture a linear continuum that runs between calm on one end and excited on the other. Again, as with attachment styles, neither state is "wrong" or "bad." There are moments to be calm and moments to be excited, moments to be low energy and moments to be high energy.

Where on this continuum, which lists some of the common signs on each side, would you place yourself right now? Yesterday? Most typically?

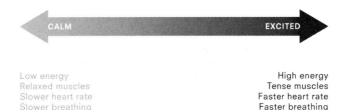

CALM   EXCITED

Low energy
Relaxed muscles
Slower heart rate
Slower breathing

High energy
Tense muscles
Faster heart rate
Faster breathing

Sherlocking

In *Wired for Dating*, Stan talks about *sherlocking* as a skill you can develop to vet a potential mate and then subsequently use as you build a long-lasting intimate partnership. Sherlocking—named for the expert detective work of Sherlock Holmes—is based on the nervous system "tells" through which we nonverbally communicate how we are doing at any given moment. These tells can provide clues about where we are on the nervous-system continuum at that moment and whether we might want to either raise or lower our energy level.

Being aware of your partner's tells is an important step to becoming experts on each other. There are probably as many tells as there are people in the world, but the tells most helpful for your work with your partner involve the face, eyes, mouth, voice, posture, and movements and gestures.

Use this "tells dictionary" to guide you as you observe your partner—and yourself:

- face
    - facial expression
    - facial coloring (pallor, blushing)
    - smile (genuine or forced)
- eyes
    - enlargement or constriction of the pupils
    - small muscle movements around the eyes
    - eye contact (avoidance of, wandering eyes, staring, present and friendly)
- mouth
    - lip corners turned up or down
    - lips relaxed or pursed
- voice
    - volume (loud or soft)
    - tone (modulated or flat)
    - laughter (giggly, raucous, sincere)
- posture
    - straight or slumped
- movements and gestures
    - fidgety and jerky or smooth and relaxed
    - foot tapping
    - hair twirling

Charlie and I have compiled our own dictionary of tells. For example, when he is bummed out, he keeps his eyes down and resists eye contact. His face loses color and becomes less animated. He also becomes more quiet in general, and when he does speak, his voice is low and soft. I often cry when I'm sad, and my face can have a droopy expression, with my lower lip protruding. On my own, I might not have noticed that about myself; however, Charlie's observations ring true for me. He also says my voice is softer and childlike, and my posture becomes more hunched when I'm feeling down. Sharing our observations with each other makes it easier to be aware of our own nervous-system tells.

Becoming Experts on Each Other

Over the next week, pay close attention to your partner's tells. Think of yourself as sherlocking—that is, playing detective with respect to your partner's tells. This will be most fun if your partner knows what you're doing and is on board with it, and even more fun if your partner is also playing detective with respect to your tells.

Here are some tips to make sure the exercise runs smoothly.

Ease into it. Start by focusing on observations of normal daily tells, rather than tells during times of high stress. You don't want to make your partner feel you're putting them under an unwanted microscope. So go slow. As you both get more comfortable with this process, add in times of stress or conflict.

Resist interpretations. This exercise can run off the rails quickly if either you or your partner make assumptions about the tells you are observing. For example, "You bit your lip; that must mean you're holding something back from me." Or "You're tapping your foot; that means you don't want to hear what I'm saying." Instead of making interpretations, check out what your partner is or was actually feeling.

Accept what you observe. At this stage, you and your partner are not trying to change or manage each other. We'll get into that later. For now, concentrate only on observing and checking out with each other what you have observed.

Compile a dictionary of tells. As you and your partner compare your sherlocking notes with one another, build a knowledge base together. Continue to observe and learn about each other. Get to the point where you can say, "When I do X, it means I'm probably feeling Y" or "When you see me do X, it probably means I need Y." In this way, you will become experts on each other.

The Coregulation Game

Once you have spent a while learning each other's tells and growing your expertise on each other, you and your partner will be ready to move into the next stage and actively help each other. This involves using both your tells and your knowledge of where you fall on the nervous-system continuum. The beauty of the mercurial quality of the nervous system is that it invites us to change or modulate it—that is, to regulate it. You can learn to regulate your own nervous system, and you and your partner can learn to help coregulate each other. I like to think of the latter as the "coregulation game." The way you play this game is to play for two winners. Your goal is to help each other move to a place on the continuum that is more comfortable for both of you.

For example, when I was in the red zone after Charlie didn't offer to get my breast pump, and my abandonment fears took over, and my nervous system shot to the excited end of the continuum, I was too agitated to think clearly. As my partner, Charlie's job was to recognize that was occurring and to soothe my nervous system and help me feel safe again. In fact, that's what ultimately happened. After I threw down the pump, I felt so ashamed at my outburst that I ran into the bedroom. Charlie followed and found me tucked in a fetal position, crying. Without saying a word, he lay down beside me and put his arms around me. Because we had done enough sherlocking and had talked about nervous-system regulation, he knew he could use his physical presence to calm me. He hugged me tightly and didn't let go. Slowly but surely, I felt myself coming back from the scary emotional place I'd just been. Once I was fully back, I was able to apologize for losing my shit, and we were able to problem solve about the pump. We also talked about how scared I was, and Charlie acknowledged he was sorry he didn't do a better job reading my tells and stopping me from sliding off into the red. Since then, we have learned to calm and soothe each other more quickly—before anyone throws anything.

Here is a framework for the coregulation game.

The coregulation game relies on teamwork. Yes, you can and should know how to regulate your own nervous system, but having your partner on your team is an extra resource. If you're feeling worked up or down in the dumps, your partner may become aware of aspects of your nervous system functioning that you are not, and they can help get you out of a rut that's harder to get out of by yourself.

Plan in advance how you and your partner will play the coregulation game. You and your partner need to learn about, discuss, and plan in advance how you want to play the coregulation game with each other. Trying to coregulate each other in the heat of the moment, without having clarified what feels good to each of you, is likely to backfire. Use the exercises in this chapter to guide you in exploration and preplanning.

Regulation needs can take different forms. Our nervous system doesn't always produce a giant explosion (as mine did); sometimes it's a more muted version of anger or excitement—for example, it might take the form of withdrawal, collapse, or shame. Most often, the coregulation game will involve one of you calming or soothing the other when they become agitated. However, there may be times when one of you has low energy, and the other can help activate that energy.

You are your partner's ally at all times. Regulating your partner's nervous system should never involve opposing or ignoring your partner's feelings. Meet your partner wherever they're at, without criticizing or finding fault. You are your partner's caretaker until they're able to think clearly again.

Calling a stop. Your partner can call a stop at any point they feel unsafe or unsure, and you must *immediately* honor that stop.

Soothe and Be Soothed

This exercise builds on the prior exercise, in which you worked on becoming experts on one another. Now you're going to embark on the coregulation game and begin to manage each other's nervous systems at times when one or both of you are stressed. As I said, the most common form of coregulation involves soothing one another, so that's what I suggest you focus on initially.

The first part in this exercise is designed to be done by you alone; it's a game of regulation solitaire. The second part is done with your partner. Ideally, your partner can also do the first part ("Soothing Yourself") before you work on the second part together.

Soothing yourself. Next time you feel stressed, take a minute to step back and notice where you are on the continuum and what specifically is happening with your nervous system. This will include some of the same kinds of tells you've already started to work with. Ask yourself:

- How slow or fast is my breath?
- What's my heart rate?
- Am I sweaty?
- Am I shaky?
- Am I flushed?
- Am I tearing up or crying?
- Do I want to curl up in a ball?
- Do I feel like lashing out?
- Do I feel like I'm sinking?

Make a list of what you notice about your nervous system. Add anything else you notice to your list.

Now explore what you can do to soothe your nervous system, to move yourself on the continuum. Here are some suggestions to consider; feel free to branch out and include whatever works best for you.

- Spend time alone.
- Get a hug from someone.
- Have a piece of chocolate.
- Exercise.
- Take a warm bath.
- Talk to a good friend.
- Meditate.
- Get a massage.
- Listen to music.

Experiment with the methods on your list and see what works best for you.

Being soothed by your partner and soothing your partner. In this step, you and your partner will play the coregulation game together. After you have both independently completed part I, compare notes and share your respective nervous-system observations. The fact that you already know many of each other's tells should help a lot.

Your purpose in sharing is to give each of you permission to step in and regulate the other's nervous system when you notice these tells in the future.

Now think about what your partner could do to soothe you. Some of these may be similar to ways you soothe yourself. Here are some ideas:

- Hold or touch you.

- Listen to you empathically.

- Repeat back to you what you're saying so you feel understood and safe.

- Give you time to be alone and regroup.

- Reassure you that everything is going to be okay.

- Help you problem solve whatever is troubling you.

- Ask you what you need most in that moment.

Finally, make an agreement about how you will play the coregulation game going forward. Your agreement might include the following:

- Grant your partner permission to help regulate your nervous system.

- Specify what means of soothing (or exciting) you welcome.

- Indicate how you will let your partner know if you want them to stop.

- Agree to stop whenever your partner requests a stop.

Tending to Your Twosome

Let me introduce you to two couples who could benefit from the ability to regulate each other's nervous systems during stressful times. For each, you will see two scenarios. In the first scenario, the partners have no awareness of their own or each other's nervous system. Their colors take over, and that's about it. In the second scenario, they are transforming themselves into experts on each other by reading their tells and managing their nervous systems. As you read, try to identify as many nervous-system tells as you can.

Alice and Brett

"So … I lost our baby," Alice says, after hanging up the phone with her doctor. Her face is pale, and her lower lip trembles as she sits on the couch and looks across the room at Brett, who is busy answering emails on his phone. "It was so hard to get pregnant in the first place. I don't think I have it in me to try again."

"Alice, you can't think that way. You have to stay strong. We'll give it another go in a couple of months." Brett looks at her briefly, then turns back to his emails. Inside, he's crushed too, but he doesn't think it would help Alice to know.

She begins to cry quietly, staring at her feet. It feels like her whole world is caving in. When she looks up and sees Brett still on his phone, she feels herself sinking even lower.

Brett senses Alice looking at him and glances up. He tells himself, *Now is not the time to be sad. I don't want to think about all the pregnancy losses we've had. I'm sick of it.*

Alice sees him looking at her and says, "What if we *never* become parents?"

That's just what Brett doesn't want to hear. "Stop it!" he snaps. "Don't even go there. We'll get pregnant again. We'll have our baby." He can feel his own distress building, so he says, "I'm going for a run. Be back in thirty or so." With that, he heads upstairs to get his running gear. His mind is racing as he laces his shoes. *I have to get out of here,* he thinks.

As he heads out the door, he gives Alice a peck on the cheek. "I love you. We'll find a way. Our baby is still out there."

Alice doesn't say anything. She sits motionless, feeling abandoned, her breathing shallow, streaks of tears on her cheeks.

♥♥♥

Pregnancy loss is hard and painful. Instead of noticing that Alice's nervous system has plummeted to the low-energy end of the continuum and that she isn't able to lift herself up, Brett focused on his own nervous system and his need to buoy himself. He forgot that she is in his care and that if her nervous system drops, their partnership tanks along with it. Let's see them try this again.

Alice's phone rings, and she sees it's her doctor. She calls out to Brett, "The doctor's calling."

He rushes over to Alice. They sit on the couch, side by side, and he reaches for her hand as she answers the phone. As Alice listens to the doctor, Brett keeps his eyes on her face. He notices her nodding, her face growing pale, and her eyes welling up with tears. He squeezes her hand to let her know he's right there with her.

"Okay. I understand," she says finally. "Thanks, doctor."

When Alice hangs up, she doesn't have to say anything, because Brett already realizes it's bad news. He turns Alice's body toward him and puts his arms around her. He knows this is what she wants him to do.

"I'm so sad," Alice says through tears.

"I know, baby. I right here with you."

They remain quietly holding each other. Brett can hear Alice crying and feel her jagged breathing. He gently rubs her back, soothing her. He feels his own anxiety and grief, but right now he's more focused on what Alice needs.

Alice feels the first big wave of emotion begin to recede. Brett's hand on her back is comforting, and she lets out a sigh as she pulls back from their embrace to look at him. She can see his eyebrows pinching, the way they do when he's holding in feelings. "I know this is hard for you too," she says.

He nods.

"Do you want to talk?" she offers.

Brett wipes a couple of tears from Alice's face. "Thanks. I'd like that. But I think I need to go for a little walk first."

"Do you want company?"

"No, thanks. I need to alone. That is, if you'll be okay for thirty minutes or so?"

"Absolutely. And if you change your mind, I'm just a text away."

♥♥♥

In this scenario, Brett leaned in to Alice's discomfort from the beginning. He took note of her tells and tended to her nervous system, meeting her where she was, without letting his own worries about their ability to become pregnant and carry a baby to term get in the way. He understood her need was greater in that moment, and there would be time for his feelings as well. Brett's support allowed Alice's grief to move through her nervous system. By regulating her nervous system, Brett helped lift Alice's energy so she could in turn support him. Being experts on each other made all the difference during a time when they both needed each other deeply.

Carlos and Steven

Carlos flies through the front door. "Stevie, I've got the best news! I'm going to be full-time faculty at the college. We're all set, babe! Health and retirement bennies and a real salary! I won't have to teach extra classes all summer, so we can actually take a vacation!"

Steven is in the kitchen making lunch. Their infant son, Ryan, is asleep in his swing by the window. "Shh!" he hisses. "You'll wake the baby."

Carlos comes barreling into the kitchen. "Kiss me! Our dreams are coming true!"

"Huh?" Steven looks up from the stove, confused. "You won a trip around the world or something?"

Carlos slows down a bit. "What do you mean, trip around the world? Didn't you hear anything I said?"

Steven frowns. "No, I didn't. I'm trying a new quick vegetarian chili recipe."

"That's nice," Carlos says in a voice that sounds clipped and irritated. His lower lip protrudes slightly, and his eyes, which were previously lit up, dim. His shoulders slump as he watches Steven stir the chili for a minute, before silently leaving the room.

"What's wrong? I thought you'd be hungry?" Steven calls after him, then adds. "What were you so excited about? Did I miss something?"

Carlos can't hear him, because he has already walked back out the front door and is sitting in his car, feeling blue.

♥♥♥

In this scenario, Steven was unable to meet and accept Carlos in his high level of excitement. Steven's inattentiveness brought Carlos down. Instead of Carlos lifting up Steven, both partners ended up alone and isolated in what could have been a moment of mutual celebration if they had drawn from their knowledge as experts on each other. Let's see them try it again.

Carlos walks in the front door, practically dancing. "Hey babe! Where are you and Ryan? I can't wait to share some good news!"

Steven leans out of the kitchen door and stage-whispers toward the entry. "We're in the kitchen. Ryan's asleep, so sneak in quietly so you can talk to me while I whip up lunch."

"Cool!" Carlos follows Steven to the stove, then puts his hands on Steven's shoulders and turns him around.

Steven sees that Carlos's eyes are twinkling with excitement. It's contagious, and he notices he's starting to feel excitement in his own chest. "So, what's going on?"

"I'm full-time faculty, babe!"

"Oh my God, congrats!" Steven plants a kiss on Carlos and gives him a giant hug. "I'm so proud of you!" He feels his own body buzzing with excitement as he looks at his love. They're both talking in whispers, but that doesn't mute the intensity of their connection.

"Thanks!" Carlos says, tearing up. "I'm so happy! I was literally jumping up and down when I got the good news. I could hardly wait to come home and tell you face to face! Seeing you look at me in this moment feels incredible. My cheeks are getting sore 'cause I'm smiling so much."

"Aww, I love you. You deserve this. And they're so lucky to have you."

"Thanks, babe."

♥♥♥

In this scenario, both men set themselves and each other up for optimum joint happiness at the excited end of the continuum. Carlos carried his excitement straight to Steven so Steven could see his tells and join him in his happiness. Steven stopped what he was doing long enough to recognize Carlos's tells and was able to meet him in his full joy. These two partners are well on their way to becoming experts on one another.

What Makes This Principle Hard?

The messaging of mainstream American popular culture can make caring for yourself and your partner challenging, especially as you enter the expecting vortex. Your twosome can seem secondary to the upcoming attraction: your baby. If you're already parents, you may just now be realizing how secondary your care, your partner's care, and the care of your relationship have become. Even without you noticing it, your relationship has been set up to play second fiddle. To practice this chapter's guiding principle, you will have to see past the cultural messaging that's coming at you from friends, family, media, and the broader society. The following are two cultural messages that can make it harder for you and your partner to care for yourselves and each other. After you read about them, see if you can think of other messages that have affected you.

Parents Are Invisible During Pregnancy

"How many weeks are you?" "Is it a boy or a girl?" "Your in-laws must be excited." "You're going to move to a better area to raise baby, right?"

Many parents-to-be (and I mean most especially moms) experience the intense mainstream cultural focus on baby as soon as they find out they are pregnant. I experienced this as full of definitive rules and precautions, all focused on the hitchhiker inside. I sometimes felt left behind as strangers offered unsolicited advice or commented on my body ("You carry high; you must be having a boy." Or "Are you sure you're not having twins?"). Everyone was more interested in my growing belly than in my mind or emotions.

When I asked my OB/GYN psychological questions about the intense emotional change that was happening, he looked confused. So I turned to some of the most widely read pregnancy literature, such as Heidi Murkoff's *What to Expect When You Are Expecting*. I didn't find much that addressed my changing internal landscape. The message I got was that it didn't matter and that I'd better focus on how to care for baby while he camped out in my belly.

This focus on baby rather than parents continues when the baby hits the scene. When a baby is born, so are parents. Yet all our language is baby centered. For example, the first three months of the baby's life are unofficially called the "fourth trimester," because babies are still changing rapidly, much as they did in the womb. They mostly eat and sleep, without much awareness that they are in this world now. But it's also the parents' first trimester of parenting. Calling it the fourth trimester reveals how our culture ignores both partners' experience of becoming parents, in all its wild and radical newness.

How can you counter this messaging? One way is to play the "*and* us too" game. You and your partner add yourselves to as many baby comments as you can. Here's an example:

A well-meaning friend asks if you guys have gotten the nursery ready for baby.

Playing the "*and* us too" game, you could say, "We're still picking out furniture for the baby's room. It's fun to set it up and get everything ready. *And* we're spending as much time as we can enjoying our family of two before she arrives."

Or your *and* could be, "We're both wrapping up career projects now."

Your *and* could be a "me too" instead of an "us too." For example, "*And* I'm spending more time in our garden in the evenings. I love to pick veggies and find new ways to prepare them."

Good Parenting Means Selflessness

"Mama, take care of your body so I can grow better." "Give your everything to the kids, they're your greatest accomplishments." "The natural state of motherhood is unselfishness." "A good dad always sacrifices his needs for our needs."

A mom-friend of mine, Tessa, told me the idea of sacrificing for baby started early for her. She had experienced depression on and off throughout her adult life and had managed it successfully with antidepressants. When she found out she was pregnant, her OB/GYN immediately suggested she wean herself from her antidepressant medication so she could "do what's best" for baby. When she asked if he could point her to research on the effect of those meds on fetuses, he only had a counter question: "Why risk it?" In that moment, Tessa felt she had become just a vehicle carrying a passenger, not a woman with a long history of depression needing care.

Fetuses are vulnerable, and pregnant women need to alter their lifestyles to best care for them. That is a fact. However, because of a cultural blind spot, not enough research has been done on all of the risks and ramifications that use of medications, alcohol, caffeine, smart phones and tablets, and exercise has on the fetus and on the mom. The conclusion, based on existing research, is simply that pregnant women should abstain from any potential risk, without consideration for their own well-being. Period. This sets up the expectation that unconditional selflessness and sacrifice are pre-reqs for the gig of parenting.

How can you counter this messaging? Here are some ways. You two give your heart, time, patience, resources, and so much more to baby. Instead of seeing that as sacrificing for baby, try honoring it and reframing it as generosity. Keep in mind that generosity is about teamwork, not competition. It doesn't require you to give more than your partner has to give, or vice versa.

You might find it helpful to visualize a generosity scale. You two must keep the scale balanced so neither is sacrificing more. If one of you feels you're being asked repeatedly to give more than you have to give, it's a team problem and needs a team solution. If your partner has tipped the scales by being especially generous, balance that out by offering them opportunities for self-care.

For example, when I was spending practically all my time at home with Jude in the early months of his life, I began to miss my pre-Jude social life. One of the ways Charlie helped me—which, in turn, helped our relationship—was suggesting I schedule more frequent hang dates sans Jude with my friends. "Frequent" was probably about twice a month, but those self-care dates buoyed me and fed my need for more adult conversation. They made me a better mom and partner.

Conclusion

Caring for yourself and for your partner is a continual journey of noticing, sherlocking, and tending to your respective nervous systems. Here we built on the attachment continuum discussed in chapter 1. Knowing and accepting where you and your partner fall on the continuum gives you a secure base for forming your partner team. In this chapter, you extended that secure base through the practice of meeting your partner where you each are on the nervous-system continuum. This tool gives you the ability to regulate each other's nervous systems and thus to function as experts on each other. In the next chapter, you'll learn about the importance of making and keeping clear agreements.

CHAPTER 3

Tightening Up Your Team

In the last two chapters, we covered a lot of ground related to the two theoretical orientations underlying this book—attachment theory and nervous-system regulation. All of this juicy information should help you dive into the nitty-gritty of launching your own tight partner team, propelled by the primary guiding principle for this book: the couple comes first. As I said in the introduction, this principle is like the oxygen mask you put on yourself before you take care of your baby—all the subsequent principles depend on that initial act of security. So the question arises: what practical strategy can you use now to stack the deck so you're more likely to put your relationship first even when life presents challenges and the going gets tough?

One immediate answer is by creating solid agreements.

Let's start by looking at some common scenarios that illustrate the effects of agreements that *don't* reflect secure functioning. Can you relate to any of these? I can relate to all of them.

On that #blessed day in July, you promised each other "till death do us part," but now you're wondering what it really meant. You're sick and tired of picking up after your partner. As you scoop up a trail of abandoned socks, you wonder, *Did I agree to be a maid when I said "I do"?* You're frustrated and resentful; just the thought of all the extra laundry and chores that will arrive with your baby bomb is enough to make you feel queasy. *Is this what commitment looks like?* you ask yourself.

Or you thought you two agreed to keep your monthly spending in check, but as you glance at your bank statement, you're annoyed to notice a bunch of charges you don't recognize that put your account in the red. You wonder if you should split up your finances or give your partner a separate account with a cap on it. You think, *I thought we were on the same page with respect to saving to buy a house. Why sabotage that with this needless spending?*

Or you're putting your relationship first but wonder if your partner got the memo. You learned their nervous system tells and are right there when they need you to provide soothing and support. Whether exciting or disappointing things happen in your life, they're the first to know. But you're waiting for your partner to step up and put the relationship first too. *Why isn't this working when I'm leading so well by example?* you wonder.

Or you and your partner are both slammed with work demands. The time to cook, clean, and take care of chores is practically nonexistent. Not to mention time for the extra emotional care you both so desperately need. You wish your partner would pull back on their career so you could dig deeper into yours, or vice versa. You think, *We should stagger our career pushes so our relationship isn't on the back burner.* You keep wanting to discuss this, but you put it off. Until one night you end up in a huge fight about how overcommitted you both are professionally, which ends without resolution. You're bummed and stressed out, and so is your partner.

Scenarios like these are common when partners don't have clear agreements with one another. When I say "agreement," I mean an agreed-upon decision you both are crystal clear on and are equally on board with. You may have an initial agreement about your long-term commitment, yet still be in the dark about what that means day to day for your party of two. How do you split up chores around the house and in the yard? Who buys the groceries? On which days do you make dinner, and when does your partner? Change diapers? You may also be unclear with respect to your mid-range agreements. For example: What are your goals as a family? Where will you go on vacations? How long do you wait before trying again to get pregnant?

It's been my observation that most couples' agreements are not as thoroughly discussed or well understood as they could be. This can set the partners up for failure. And when you throw a baby into the mix, with all the increased responsibilities that come with a newborn, the need for clear, thoughtful agreements becomes all the more critical.

The principle I cover in this chapter will guide you and your partner to make agreements that support your decision to put your coupledom first. I begin by discussing the foundational agreement you and your partner can make to tighten up your team. Then we look at how you can honor, respect, and build upon your initial agreement on a day-to-day basis.

Guiding Principle 3: You and your partner make agreements with each other that you respect.

When you and your partner decide to invite a baby into your party of two—and truly speaking, even before you reach that juncture—you can't rely on honeymoon-style romance to be the impetus for your showing up for your relationship. You have to show up even when you're tired, cranky, hungry, frustrated, or overwhelmed. And you have to do it because this is what you agreed to, knowing you are stronger and happier together when you function securely as a team.

Yet managing to show up at each and every necessary moment can be a tricky business for couples. Witness the four scenarios I just described. Consider what went wrong in each.

- The partner left picking up socks is experiencing a disconnect between an initial agreement to care for each other and what happens in the details of each moment. The same can be said for the partner leaving socks scattered about. Both members of this team need some guidelines to help them feel respected, cared for, and secure.

- In the case of the busted finances, the two partners have different interpretations of their agreement—if they even have an agreement. The disappointed partner is troubleshooting solo, and the it's-raining-money partner isn't considering the consequences of overspending. These two need to concretize their financial agreement and then respect and abide by it.

- The partner working hard to put the relationship first is doing so in the absence of a clear team agreement and without communication about what constitutes welcomed support. The other half, who didn't get the memo and isn't picking up any tells, is equally responsible for this communication mishap. Both partners don't realize the shared, mutual responsibility on which agreements are based.

- The overworked partners don't appreciate the value of ongoing communication about their agreements. Their attachment colors are large and in charge, keeping them from talking about their family's needs. Even if both silently wish for change, neither is able to initiate it by bringing up a potentially difficult conversation.

These scenarios highlight some of the key ingredients that can go a long way toward ensuring agreements don't go awry: respect, mutuality, and clear and direct communication. Both team members need to know what is expected of them and what to expect from their partner. This clarity creates security.

You can kick-start your winning team by creating a strong foundational agreement to put your partnership first. In *Wired for Love*, Stan talks about operationalizing secure functioning by making a pact to put your relationship first. That pact is your bedrock, your ground zero. It is a living agreement you and your partner continue to come back to. At the same time, you can continually reinforce and tighten it, as well as make additional agreements in response to what comes at you during the course of daily life. If you want to reap the benefits of the secure-functioning team you're creating, then respecting the agreements you make with each other needs to become a daily practice.

Three practical tools can support you and your partner to make successful agreements with each other: (1) your foundational couple agreement, (2) making and respecting your agreements as a daily practice, and (3) circling back to your agreements in times of stress. Let's look at each of these.

Your Foundational Couple Agreement

You and your partner may be making a formal agreement for the first time as you read this book. Or you might be adding to vows you've already made or vows you plan to make at an upcoming commitment ceremony. Even if you've made a formal agreement before, you will want to revisit it now as parents or as you become parents. As parents, you don't have the luxury of skating by on implicit or unconscious agreements. You want it clear, explicit, and in writing.

Both you and your partner have to know what you are agreeing to and be on board with the agreement for it to work. If you have agreements that are unsaid and implicit, you won't know what is expected for your band to rock and roll. And you won't know how to handle accountability when one of you inevitably misses band practice. If an agreement is murky, it sets both partners up for failure. Even if it's explicit and carefully thought out, if one partner is all-in and the other is not, the all-in partner can end up feeling hurt, resentful, and underappreciated.

The purpose of your foundational agreement is to guide you in putting your coupledom first and setting up the expectation that you will relate to one another with respect, mutuality, and clear and direct communication. Exactly how your agreement is worded should be unique to your relationship. I offer the following ingredients just to get your juices flowing. Feel free to pick and choose among them and to add your own as you come up with the recipe for your own agreement.

- We agree to have each other's backs.

- We agree to be partners in crime.

- We agree to be in each other's care.

- We agree to share our inner worlds with each other.

- We agree to provide each other with shelter from the storm.

- We agree to be friends in the darkness and in the light.

- We agree to be each other's suns, around which we orbit.

- We agree to be each other's number one fan.

- We agree to give each other total freedom to be ourselves.

- We agree to protect each other in public and in private.

AGREEING TO PUT YOUR RELATIONSHIP FIRST

The purpose of this exercise is to create an agreement that articulates the foundation of your couple team. You should both gain clarity about what you want your relationship to look and feel like and about what behaviors are okay and not okay.

1. Carve out some uninterrupted couple time when both of you are rested (as rested as possible if you're already parents and continually fatigued) and undistracted. You may need several uninterrupted sessions to flesh out your agreements post-baby.

2. Discuss with your partner what it means to each of you to put the relationship first. As a starting point, you can use my sample agreement ingredients, but don't be limited to those. Your agreement can have as many or as few parts as you choose.

3. Discuss the pros and cons of each ingredient so you both fully understand what you are agreeing to and why. This makes you both equally responsible for your side of the agreement.

4. When you're ready, both of you should be able to state your agreement and why you agree to it. Put it in writing. Hang it on your refrigerator, on your bedroom wall, or in a sacred space. One day you may want to tell your child about your agreement and explain that they can count on you to practice it every day.

5. Your couple agreement should be alive. People and situations change, so as needed, revise and update it so it serves you better. Check in with your partner regularly about how they're experiencing your agreement. Discussing how you both feel about it, including the security it offers, brings your agreement to life.

Agreements as a Daily Practice

When Charlie and I were struggling as a couple post–baby bomb, I recalled Stan's recommended couple pact. It occurred to me that might be just what we needed in the moment. So I suggested to Charlie that we make a new pinky swear pact to one another to help us get back on track as a team. He was immediately in. We had made an agreement pre-Jude to put our relationship first and had defined what that meant for us then, as a twosome. But after we became parents and faced a new set of challenges, we needed to revisit that foundational agreement, redefine it, and then recommit.

Our new pact gave us the secure base we needed to thrive as a family of three. But as solid and dependable as that base was, we quickly discovered it was no longer enough to have a single, one-size-fits-all couple agreement. We faced a seemingly endless wellspring of opportunities to make agreements—big and small. Not only that, but for those agreements to be meaningful, we had to continually demonstrate that we were doing everything we could to uphold them and that we fully respected them. Before long, making and respecting our agreements had become a daily practice for us.

By "daily practice," I don't mean we scheduled an hour a day to sit down and discuss our agreements. Far from it! What I mean is that we brought a 24/7 awareness of our agreements to all aspects of our lives. That awareness led us to new agreements. For example, we committed to being available to each other throughout each day, to tracking each other's highs and lows, to giving each other lots of hugs and smiles and physical touch, and to sharing a bedtime ritual each evening.

It can be easy to overlook this kind of regular practice. You can become lulled into believing the agreement you inked many moons ago will carry you through thick and thin. In our busy modern world, it's easy to forget that commitments are living, breathing things that require active daily participation. Add a baby to boot, and it's even more imperative to practice daily respect for your couple agreements.

When you and your partner approach making and respecting your agreements as a daily practice, you no longer let things slide under the rug because they're too hard to deal with. Instead, at the slightest sign of trouble, you check in with yourself and each other to see how whatever is happening in the moment relates to your relevant existing agreements. You ask three basic questions:

- Does our agreement cover this situation?

- If it does, are we respecting our agreement?

- If it doesn't, do we need a new agreement here?

Having clarified these questions, you can figure out what you need to do to show respect, to refine an existing agreement, or to form a new one.

Here's what two of our earlier problem scenarios might look like if the partners (I'll give them names) made respecting their agreements a daily practice.

Nona: (putting irritation aside, based on her belief they can work this out) Hey Clay, about those socks of yours ….

Clay: Socks? (Catching Nona's I-mean-business tone, as well as the slight twinkle in her eye.) Yeah, right, sorry about that. I know we made an agreement to both be responsible for picking stuff up.

Nona: Glad to hear you remember and that you're sorry. But you gotta know this isn't working for me. I can't be your maid. I think we need a new agreement.

Clay: Babe, I totally don't want you to feel like a maid. But honestly, I don't think we need a new agreement. I just need to fully respect the agreement we already have.

Nona: Can you do that?

Clay: I can. And if I don't, I'll be the first to take responsibility for saying we need to redefine our agreements about household chores.

In this scenario, notice how the partners communicate rather than stay isolated in their own bunkers. Nona is able to bring up the issue without exploding at Clay, because they've already established basic ground rules. As it turns out, Clay is aware of their agreement, so the most logical first action is to step up his respect for it. You get the sense that their process started with some mutual agreements and continues as a daily practice as they both work to make good on their commitments.

Let's look at a second scenario—our partners with the financial issues.

Tim: Max, is this a good moment for us to talk?

Max: I just finished the dishes, so sure.

Tim: (as they get comfortable on the couch) I need to tell you that I was so upset earlier when I discovered those big charges on our account.

Max: I'm glad you're mentioning it. But I'm a bit surprised. I told you a while ago I was upgrading my workstation. I also said I'd book that weekend we talked about.

Tim: Yeah, I guess I knew about those things. But I didn't realize they were all coming together this month.

Max: I didn't know you didn't realize that.

Tim: (laughing) I guess we both made some assumptions.

Max: I guess so. I can look into cancelling the weekend getaway. I don't think it's too late for a refund.

Tim: No, no, please don't. I'm looking forward to getting away, just the two of us. In fact, I was planning to book it soon and surprise you.

Max: Okay. Sounds like we were both trying to surprise each other. That's cool. (*Leans in and kisses Tim, then stops abruptly.*) But I think we need to sit down and go over financial stuff so we can make an agreement that works for both of us.

Here, the partners quickly realize they lack a clear agreement that covers all bases when it comes to their finances. They may have talked about their spending, but they aren't clear about how much money, when it will be spent, or who's going to spend it. The fact that they have embarked on a daily practice of respecting their agreements allows them to pinpoint the issues without too much delay and to quickly set about fixing things. It's all a work in progress!

Your Inventory of Agreements

You will note I'm not talking here about the in-the-weeds decision-making you and your partner will have to engage in to iron out agreements in an ongoing way. That's the focus of the guiding principle in the next chapter. For now, let's keep the focus on the daily practice of making and respecting your agreements. To do this, it's helpful to keep an inventory of the aspects of your relationship that stand to benefit from agreements.

First, let's compile some common categories for which you and your partner may need agreements to achieve maximum team tightness:

- careers

- childrearing

- household management

- finances

- vacations

- friends and community

- romance

Your daily practice will involve maintaining an awareness of the agreements you have in these areas—or in other areas you identify with your partner. For example, if you find yourselves both slammed with work, you might stop to consider any agreements you've made related to careers. Or if you're tussling over your child's potty training, you'd consider your agreements related to childrearing.

This list is intentionally broad to give you room to create your own inventory, tailored to your relationship. Here are more specific items to keep in mind as you and your partner create your list. You can see these both as ingredients for your broader agreements and as checkpoints to see how well you're respecting those agreements:

- how available we are to each other throughout the day

- who initiates discussions, and about what topics

- who takes the lead on laundry, dishes, and other chores

- known areas of disagreement

- what we share well and what we don't

LAUNCHING YOUR DAILY PRACTICE OF AGREEMENTS

At some point after you and your partner have created your foundational agreement and have gained a sense of how it's working for you, sit down again. This time, discuss how you will work with the agreements you make going forward. You can think of this as launching your daily practice because, unlike your foundational agreement, your new agreements will involve an ongoing process of assessment, clarification, and revision. Of course, you'll want to revisit your foundational agreement as well, but I wouldn't expect you to do that on a daily basis.

During your discussion, consider these questions:

- Are we both on the same page with our agreements?

- Do we both know what's expected of us?

- Do we know what's expected of each other?

- What new or revised agreements do we (or will we) want to make?

- How (and when) do we want to check in with each other about our agreements?

Circling Back

We've been talking about using agreements to become a tight team of partners who always put your coupledom first. But what happens in those moments when it doesn't work to put the couple first? For example, you're in the midst of negotiating family business with your partner, and one of you receives an unexpected call you need to take. Or you're so deep in a discussion about whether to try IVF or adopt that you've lost track of time, and now the friends who were coming over for dinner are knocking at the door. As a party of two, you've undoubtedly faced plenty of such times. And I promise you'll face infinitely more when you become a party of three. Every parent has experienced the baby or child interruption. And we all know that sometimes baby's needs *do* have to come first. At those times, you and your partner need a contingency plan that allows you to shelve whatever is happening between you so you can tend to baby.

The key is not to let the need to shelve conversations undermine your couple agreements. You might be tempted to say, "We failed" or "Our agreement to put our partnership first works sometimes but not always." No. Your foundational agreement and all your other agreements have to be solid enough to incorporate times when you need to put baby first. Or job first. Or sick grandma first. Or when one partner absolutely needs alone time.

Circling back is the tool you can use to do this. Specifically, it is a skill involving five steps. Note that these steps include an agreement that, like the agreements we've been discussing, must be mutual.

1. Notice that your conversation with your partner must end for the time being due to baby's needs or because something else has taken precedence.

2. Signal to your partner that the conversation must end.

3. Make a quick verbal agreement to circle back when you guys can.

4. Both of you acknowledge the end for now.

5. Circle back and resume your conversation at a later time.

Both of you are responsible for circling back. It could be later that day, the next day, or next week. Unless it involves a time-sensitive issue, it doesn't matter when the conversation is picked up; what matters is that you both agree to do so and check in with each other about when. The goal is that no conversation, issue, need, or want is dropped entirely. Successful circling back creates a feeling of goodwill and confidence between you.

Here's how it works for Sarah and Lucas. Sarah is seven months pregnant and is worried their apartment will soon be too small. She explains her concern to Lucas over scones and coffee. "If we're going to take care for ourselves as a couple, like we agreed, having enough space is important. It might sound like a luxury, but it's not."

"I hear what you're saying," Lucas says, "but the thought of moving before River is born makes me nervous."

"It'll be easier now than trying to juggle everything when we're parents," Sarah argues. "I know you—you'll go crazy if we lose our home work space, which is a given if we stay here."

Lucas glances at his phone. "I want to keep hashing this out, Sarah, but if I don't leave in five, I'll be late for a staff meeting."

It's already hard juggling stuff now—just imagine what's in store, Sarah thinks. But she understands that he needs to leave now. "Okay. I was going to look at apartment listings today, but I'll hold off till we have a chance to talk more. Do you think we can circle back this evening?"

Lucas hesitates. He puts on his jacket, then says, "Moving is a big deal time-wise and money-wise. I need to give this some thought."

"Take your time, babe," Sarah says. "If you're not ready to discuss it tonight, that's okay. Just tell me, and we'll circle back later."

During the day, Sarah starts to feel anxious about the lack of clarity on their housing situation. In spite of her promise to hold off on looking for a new apartment, she goes online to check listings. But immediately she stops. *We made an agreement to take care of ourselves as a couple, and if I do this now, I'm putting my needs first. I'm going against our agreement.*

That evening, as Lucas and Sarah sit down for dinner, he brings up the possibility of moving. "I thought about it during my break this afternoon, and I think you're onto something. I get how beneficial it would be to have enough space, especially when River's here. I'm just not sure the timing works."

"In the end, I think it'll be worth it," Sarah says. "But you're right, the thought of planning a move at seven-months preggers is a bit crazy." She reaches across the table and takes Lucas's hand. "I didn't realize how stressful becoming parents could be. I just want us to be as prepared as possible."

"I'm stressed too, love," Lucas says. "But I'm confident we're going to figure all this out. We have each other. We're a solid team."

Sarah lets out a sigh. "I'm glad you circled back tonight. This would be so much harder if I was stuck in my own head, wondering if you were even willing to discuss it."

Lucas squeezes her hand. "Don't ever doubt that I'm willing to discuss whatever you're feeling. As long as we keep talking to each other, we'll be fine."

Sarah nods. "And I'm fine if we don't reach a decision tonight. Maybe we can set a time frame for ourselves. Say, agree to make a decision by the end of this week?"

"Works for me!" Lucas beams. "If we circle back one or two times, I think we'll know what works best for our family."

♥♥♥

At this point, both partners are pleased to be upholding their agreement to take care of each other as they plan for the needs of their family, on their way to becoming a party of three. In fact, after baby arrives, circling back becomes an even more important practice for couples. The kinds of interruptions you face as a twosome—leaving for work, taking an important phone call, and so on—are much more predictable than the interruptions that occur with a baby. You never know when baby will wake up or demand attention, forcing you to abort an important conversation.

What Makes This Principle Hard?

This may be the first time you've considered the importance of creating and making agreements with your partner. I'm sure you two have figured things out together, but this principle goes beyond that. I'd like to cover two obstacles so you're fully equipped to practice this principle with flying colors. One is a lack of personal modeling, the other is cultural.

You've Never Seen Couples Doing This

"My parents didn't have explicit agreements, so why should I?" "My mom was the boss in our house growing up, so I figured I'd defer to my wife." "Couples do that? Sounds like a lot of work!"

It's hard to imagine, let alone do, something you haven't seen done before. I can relate to this personally. Growing up, I don't remember my parents explicitly making and respecting agreements. I'm sure they had agreements, but these weren't part of our family culture, and they didn't model the practice for us kids. So when I first learned about couple pacts from Stan, I thought, *Tell me more!* It was bit like imagining that I was Oz, able to see everything behind the curtain. The idea of being able to create and respect agreements was intriguing but also foreign. If this is you too, don't worry! You and your partner can be trailblazers for your family. Here's how to get started.

Acknowledge this is new and be gentle with yourself and your partner. Being gentle is generally a good practice, but it's especially important when you're experimenting with new things and growing together. Growth and change can create a feeling of vulnerability, and the best way to support yourself and your partner is to realize and respect that. Be gentle as you create your foundational couple agreement, and continue that tenderness as you negotiate additional agreements.

Congratulate each other for each new agreement. I'm a firm believer in the power of celebrating wins, even if they're small. You will find it easier to bring up new areas for agreement if you've fully appreciated the success of your foundational couple agreement. That might be as simple as high fiving each other or something more celebratory.

Model agreements for your kids. Bring your kids on your trailblazing path with you! As I suggested, you may want to share your initial couple agreement with your kid(s) so they can count on you both to practice it daily. The same goes for additional agreements. As your children age, and when your couple agreements are age appropriate, share them so your children know this is a crucial part of partnering and are better equipped for their own future relationships.

Cultural Gender Roles Dictate Agreements

"Most of the time, he's pretty good at helping me with the kids." "I'm lucky he works to support me staying home with the kids." "I don't know where the sunscreen is. Ask your mom."

Cultural gender roles, as exemplified by these quotes, can create default agreements about who's responsible for doing what. Instead of making conscious agreements, you go with what you think is expected or what feels customary. This kind of cultural power is pervasive. In my experience, parenthood tends to intensify gender roles, with mothers becoming the default primary parent. It's fine if you and your partner prefer that path, but if it's not a conscious and mutual agreement, you're likely asking for trouble down the line. A mom-friend of mine was the permanent nighttime parent in her family by default, because she had nursed each child. One day, she realized this and decided she wanted a change. So she and her partner came up with a new agreement that split their responsibility for nighttime parenting. And they didn't stop there. Now they actively look for ways culture has influenced their parenting roles. Here are some ways to counter that messaging.

Become aware of default agreements based on cultural norms. You and your partner can make it a game to notice ways in which you are unconsciously influenced by cultural expectations. Give yourselves permission to ham it up a bit as you break free from these expectations and make more conscious choices for your partnership. ("Let me clear the table, dear. I'd hate for you to strain yourself after working all day, bringing home the bacon." Or "I can't believe the house isn't sparkling. What did you do all day?") In this situation, a little humor is better than piling up resentment.

Create housework and child-rearing responsibility lists. Now that you guys have created a little levity about the culture's impact on your partnership, it's time to get to the business of changing it. Together, compile a list of all your family's shared duties. To truly change your family culture, you need to make this list together—it's not a mom job—and then tackle it together. Go through the list with your partner and delegate each responsibility, based not on gender but on what works best for your family. You may want to consider interest, time availability, and skill level. Once you two have decided who's doing what, when, and how often, make an agreement to solidify it. Adjust accordingly, as interests and availability change.

Conclusion

One way to ensure that you and your partner function as a solid team is to cocreate a living agreement to put your relationship first. This can include being direct, protecting each other in public and in private, valuing each other's perspectives and needs, and treating each other with respect and kindness. Your couple agreement provides a secure foundation, which you then bolster through a daily practice of being aware of the status of your agreements, respecting them, and revising them whenever needed. You also need a contingency plan so you don't forsake your agreements whenever life intervenes and work, baby, or something else needs to take precedence. In such situations, circling back allows you to shelve a conversation so you can attend to the matter at hand and then return to it later.

In the next chapter, we move on to your party of three, starting with life as an expecting couple. We'll also build on our discussion about couple agreements by focusing on how you and your partner can best go about making decisions together—both the many decisions that arise while expecting your little buddy and those you face when your buddy is already here.

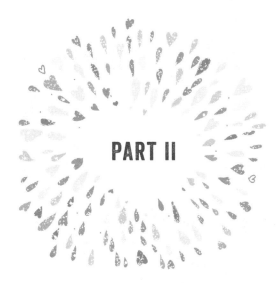

PART II

Two Become
Three

CHAPTER 4

Expecting and Beyond

Tokiko and Naomi sit across from Tokiko's parents at the restaurant and excitedly announce, "We're pregnant!"

"Oh my! Congrats!" Tokiko's mom says, as her eyes water.

"Fantastic!" her dad chimes in.

Tokiko and Naomi glance at each other, relieved. They've been on a fertility journey for years but telling Tokiko's parents is huge. For as long as Tokiko can remember, her parents wanted her to marry a "nice Japanese American man." It was hard telling them she'd found a lovely Caucasian American woman to settle down with. But they've come around to love Naomi and respect Tokiko's choices as a queer woman.

"We're happy you're happy," Naomi says.

"We're finally going to be grandparents!" Tokiko's mom says, then turns to her daughter. "I trust you've got the best medical care lined up?"

Relieved her mother isn't being her usual critical self, Tokiko says, "Of course, Mom," then offers casually, "After endless rounds of IVF, I'm tired of being poked and prodded. I'm thinking of getting a midwife for a home birth."

Naomi looks stunned, but Tokiko doesn't notice any of her tells.

"Without any poking, you wouldn't be pregnant." Tokiko's mom frowns, then looks at her husband. "Your dad and I won't let you take any unreasonable risks with our precious baby."

Tokiko's dad is nodding agreement. "Have you consulted your brother? He's a surgeon, but I'm sure he knows the best OB/GYNs in this area."

Naomi shifts in her chair. This is a conversation she expected to have with Tokiko alone. *Having a home birth is news to me*, she thinks. *We've hardly begun to talk about birth plans.* She feels her face reddening with irritation but remains silent, hoping Tokiko will step in to challenge her parents.

And she does. "Mom, Dad, please don't worry. I've got this handled."

"But—" her mom says.

Her dad puts a hand on his wife's arm, signaling that he wants to keep the peace. "Tokiko," he says, "as soon as you find out if it's a boy or a girl, tell us, so we can buy the right clothes and toys. And, of course, we want to be with you on the big day."

"You'll be the first to know everything," Tokiko says, glad not to argue but forgetting she and Naomi haven't made decisions about any of this.

But Naomi hasn't forgotten, and hearing Tokiko's parents will be at the birth puts her over the edge. "I don't know why I'm here!" she bursts out. "You three are making all the decisions about the birth of our child without me. What am I, the token wife?" With that, she pushes back her chair and rushes off to the restroom.

Tokiko is left alone with her parents. *Such a big baby, running away and embarrassing me like this,* she thinks, her face flushed with anger. *What the heck's wrong with me talking to my parents? I'm the one who's pregnant.*

♥♥♥

In previous chapters, we talked about the importance of being a partner team and putting your relationship first, including making strong couple agreements. But it's one thing to make agreements and another to implement them in each new hot situation that arises. In fact, when you decide to expand your family into a party of three, you may find yourselves entering an "expecting vortex." Suddenly, you're bombarded with so many decisions that you can lose sight of your agreements, and even of what it means to be secure functioning. You forget to work as a team and to consult each other.

The guiding principle in this chapter focuses on the key skill of decision-making. First I give you a process you can use to make decisions—both while expecting and beyond. The second part of the chapter covers decision-making for you as parents more broadly, including how to function as a two-person "insider" team while consulting others for their expertise and experience.

Guiding Principle 4: You and your partner make decisions as a team.

Parenting is one of the first high-stakes projects many couples undertake together. Maybe you and your partner collaborated on setting up your home or planning your wedding, but that's nothing compared with expecting and then raising a person. So it's natural to experience some growing pains and shifting of perspectives while homing in on the best ways to work with each other on this epic endeavor.

Day in and day out, you face decisions—some big, others small. Some may involve implementing agreements you've already forged, others may serve as the groundwork for new agreements. Think of all these choices as weaving the fabric of your life together. The decisions you make today become your life tomorrow, and if you follow a collaborative process to make them, you'll build a deep sense of trust in one another that allows you to make decisions with greater and greater ease.

To consider how things can go awry when couples don't make decisions as a team, let's get back to Naomi and Tokiko. Even if they briefly discussed birth plans, they never came close to settling on one. At the restaurant, Tokiko got carried away with baby excitement and jitters and didn't stop to consult Naomi about any of the decisions her parents were pushing. To make matters worse, Naomi didn't have an effective way of reminding Tokiko that she was a co-captain of their team. Let's revisit this scenario and see how their dinner could go with both women acting as decision-making team players.

On their way to the restaurant, Tokiko and Naomi discuss how they can support each other as they spill the news to Tokiko's parents. They decide to hold hands as they announce their pregnancy and to monitor each other's nervous-system tells, especially during tense moments. Naomi reminds Tokiko they haven't yet fully discussed their birth plan or who'll be present at the birth, and Tokiko agrees not to get into any of that tonight. Both women are clear about what they want to share and what they want to keep to themselves.

After they share the news—holding hands and saying in unison, "We're pregnant!"—Tokiko's mom says, "I trust you've got the best medical care lined up?"

"We love your concern, Mom. Naomi and I are just getting organized, but we got this. Please give us a little time."

Naomi squeezes Tokiko's hand underneath the table, signaling she's proud of Tokiko for putting down that boundary.

"Okay," Tokiko's mom says, then launches into a series of questions: "How far along are you? Are you feeling okay? Eating well?"

Tokiko turns toward Naomi, and the two women connect through eye contact for a moment. Naomi understands that, as they discussed earlier,

Tokiko wants her to play an active role in the discussion. She says, "Tokiko is fourteen weeks pregnant. She's feeling great. We're in the process of building our birth team. We'll keep you posted, I promise."

Tokiko's dad makes a toast, "To our baby … uh … what's the gender? Do you know?"

Tokiko says, "We don't. Naomi and I need to talk more about this, and we may want to keep it a surprise."

Tokiko's parents look a little sad, so Naomi jumps in to reassure them: "I think you'll be awesome grandparents to either a boy or a girl, so we're covered either way."

Tokiko smiles, grateful for Naomi's help.

Tokiko's dad senses his daughter's happiness in her partnership and says, "This child is lucky to have you both as moms."

♥♥♥

In this take two, Naomi and Tokiko teamed up ahead of time, which resulted in overall ease and fluidity over dinner, even during clunky moments. They know they still have work to do about some important issues, but that didn't lessen their team spirit. Compared with take one, their commitment to respecting each other as the co-captains of their family ship made a big difference in how they were with one another and also how they presented themselves to Tokiko's parents. It's possible the strength of their team rippled out to Tokiko's parents and helped them respect Naomi and Tokiko's decisions.

Co-captains of Your Family Ship

Having agreed to put your coupledom first, it still takes practice to remember you two are a team—not you and your mom or you and this book; you and your partner! What follows is a process you can use, as co-captains of your family ship, to navigate the decisions that face you and to do so as a secure-functioning team. This is the process Charlie and I use. We've discovered that teaming up on the big decisions has given us greater trust and confidence and has made smaller, everyday decisions almost effortless.

If you are currently expecting, you can apply this process to your immediate decisions. If baby is already with you, use it for decisions relevant now. Later in the chapter, we'll discuss how this decision-making process applies to different phases of parenthood.

This decision-making process can be broken down into eight steps:

1. Alert your partner that you'd like to make a decision together. One of you may naturally be what I call the "initiator of change" in your family. The initiator has the big ideas and may have initiated a commitment or suggested expanding your tribe. However, for decision-making in general, both partners need to take responsibility for alerting each other.

2. Do some individual thinking and researching so you come to your meeting well informed. While you can begin by gathering advice from trusted people and resources, ultimately it's up to you two to talk it out and decide what's best for your family.

3. Schedule a time that works for both of you to sit down and discuss the pending decision. Meet in a place where you can limit distractions and be fully present with the process. Turn off those cell phones!

4. Sit face to face. This will help you stay in real time and be attuned to each other's nervous systems during the conversation. Some couples like to walk and talk. If you do this, pause frequently to look at each other and do a visual scan to pick up any nonverbal tells.

5. Articulate the decision to be made. Make sure you are on the same page with respect to the decision you want to make.

6. Share your respective ideas. Take turns speaking and listening as you each share your thoughts about what could constitute the best decision.

7. Futurize about how each possible decision might play out. By "futurize," I mean imagine what your life could look like in the future if you pursue a particular course. Consider all the practical as well as long-term implications—all the "what-ifs." Futurizing helps weed out obvious wrong choices for your family.

8. Stay engaged until you arrive at a decision together. This may require multiple talks. Don't rush it! If you don't have an immediate chance to reconvene, hold off on making the decision until you can talk more.

When I was pregnant, one big decision Charlie and I made together was picking our baby's name. It was a fun, creative process involving research and lots of futurizing. We had multiple hangs to hash it out. The first was right after we left the doctor's appointment where we learned we were having a boy. In this case, we had time to go to a restaurant for a late breakfast; we didn't need to schedule anything.

We sat face to face and confessed we both had already been considering names. I had my favs and Charlie had his, and they couldn't have been more different. I can be a bit the bossy pants when I'm anxious. Knowing I can fall into that non-team-like behavior, Charlie reached across the table to hold my hand and said, "Don't worry. We'll find the perfect name for our son. Let's start a Google doc."

I laughed. Never had I imagined a doc could turn into something so romantic!

During our next hang, armed with a doc titled THE BOY, we decided that both of us had equal nix power. This allowed for some quick edits (sorry, Wren, Dion, and Elliot). I pushed hard for Lucas, but Charlie wasn't feeling it. He let me keep it in our doc for a while and humored all my Lucas-is-an-awesome-name selling points, but ultimately he levied his nix power. We used futurizing to envision how our son might feel with one or another name. Because we were giving him Charlie's last name, we wanted to make sure his maternal family was represented too, which took some fine-tuning. When I was about ready to pop, we decided on Jude Nelson, with Nelson coming from my side of the family.

We also faced a follow-up decision: whether to keep the baby's name secret. I leaned toward sharing it, and Charlie leaned toward privacy. I'm a big sharer of things, and he's a big keeper of things, so that was no surprise. However, futurizing brought clarity for both of us when Charlie said, "What if we tell your mom, and she's not enthusiastic? What if we pick up doubt from people whose opinions we value, and then we second-guess our choice?" We decided to put Jude's name into a vault until he was here.

I'm glad we spent the time hashing this out and learning from each other. The moment of introducing Jude to my mom in person wouldn't have turned out so perfectly if Charlie and I hadn't engaged in this decision-making process together.

Bring Secure Functioning to Decisions

As co-captains, you and your partner will be most successful with the decision-making process if you operate from a stance of secure functioning. This means bringing the qualities of openness, transparency, mutuality, equal collaboration, and respect.

Start the process by agreeing to be open about your preferences, opinions, and knowledge or lack thereof. When everything is on the table, neither of you has to guess what the other wants, doesn't want, or doesn't care about. For example, I told Charlie upfront it was important to me to raise a feminist and that my side of the family be represented in our son's name. Of course, being transparent doesn't mean your partner will acquiesce to whatever you want; it simply means you won't hit each other with big surprises down the line.

You also commit to being equally educated about each decision. Each of you is responsible for thinking critically, doing the necessary research, and gathering advice and ideas from friends and family. This might sound like lots of work, and it is! But the payoff—which you'll both collect—is the creation of a secure-functioning team. When done successfully, making decisions as a team fosters deeper trust. When done poorly or not at all, partners can accrue resentment and a go-it-alone attitude.

You may not agree with what your partner thinks is best, but you need to respect it. When Charlie and I sat down to discuss our ideas about going public with our chosen name, we each listened with respect, not saying anything that could have led the other to feel their views were wrong or silly. Our mutual respect allowed us to weigh all our feelings, priorities, and needs. And respect breeds greater transparency. Many partners shut down sharing their opinions because they have experienced their point of view being minimized, disregarded, shamed, or criticized. A secure-functioning team is built by respecting and trying to understand each other's perspectives.

Making Team Decisions While Expecting

Expanding your family presents an infinite array of decisions to be made. With each, you will find input coming at you from so many sources: doctors, midwives, doulas, your parents and in-laws, sisters, brothers, your friends who are parents, strangers, and even books. It's natural to feel vulnerable and uncertain at this time and to be forgetful of your partner team. You may be reading this right now and thinking, *Uh-oh, I didn't remember to ask my partner before I decided to potty train our daughter.* Or *I have to make all these pregnancy-related decisions alone because my partner isn't really available.* As we've discussed, powerful cultural messaging can discourage couples from acting as a team. Decision-making is no exception. So don't beat yourself up if you have learning to do in this arena.

Let's start by looking at some of the decisions facing expecting or hope-to-be-expecting parents. Tokiko and Naomi's decision was about their birth plan, and I shared the example of Charlie and I picking a name. Of course, your first decision was whether to have a child—which you may or may not have made intentionally or together. Here's a sampling of other key decisions:

- when to begin trying to conceive

- whether to adopt

- whether to use a surrogate

- whether to tell family if you are using donor sperm or eggs

- whether both partners go to doctor and midwife appointments together

- gender reveal

- whether to breastfeed or use formula

- sleeping arrangements

- maternity and paternity leave

- childcare

- birth control

Please add to the list as you work through this book. And feel free to make notes in your journal.

Some of these decisions (e.g., breastfeeding, childcare, birth control options) are obviously made postpartum. You won't know, for example, if you'll be able to nurse until you try. However, beginning to discuss these decisions, doing your research, and getting thoughts and feelings on the table before baby arrives will give you a head start. And you'll both have to practice flexibility, because in the fluid lives of expecting parents, decisions are rarely hard and fast. Odds are you won't make a birth plan that requires no adaptation. There are way too many variables. So I encourage you to talk about your backup plans. That way, you'll have some ideas up your sleeve that you two can bust out when the unexpected happens.

Making Team Decisions as Parents

When your baby bomb goes off, your family leaps from two to three (or more), and you have a zillion new decisions to make, it can be hard to follow the first guiding principle: the couple comes first. I like to look at parental decision-making from the perspective of insiders and outsiders. You two are the insiders in all your glory as co-captains of your family ship. Everyone else is an outsider. Including your child.

Putting your couple first is like creating a magical, invisible force field around the two of you. This field gives you security and strength and an ever-present sense of loving protection. From this safe and secure place, you can reach out and incorporate others (the outsiders) in whatever ways you choose. And yet you two always return to your insider circle, your coupledom.

We saw the role of outsiders with Tokiko and Naomi. Tokiko's mistake was bringing her parents (outsiders) into decisions she and Naomi (insiders) needed to first discuss alone. This illustrates the importance of insiders making sure outsiders don't hijack the decision-making process. This doesn't mean making team decisions as parents is all about holding your outsiders at bay. In fact, outsiders have important roles to play. The key is to maintain your status as insiders while allowing support from outsiders. When you put the security of your partnership at the forefront, you can relax, knowing that neither of you will be blindsided by a decision an outsider was allowed to make. This culti-vates trust, ease, and creativity in your parenting and partnering. Let's look at some ways this can play out.

Asserting Insider Status

When Jude was about six months, I was nursing on demand every night. I was exhausted to the point that my fatigue was affecting my mental and physi-cal health. I couldn't even see that we needed a solution. Moreover, I had a strong outsider voice in my head: our pediatrician had suggested Jude be breast-fed until one year old. I knew Dr. Woods was an outsider, but I put a lot of weight on his word. I was concerned that if I stopped nursing on demand, my milk supply would go down, and I wouldn't make it to one year.

Charlie took the lead in asserting our insider status by initiating a discussion. As I was coming downstairs after putting Jude down for a nap, he called out, "Hey love, I'd like to talk to you."

I made my way over to the couch, where he was beckoning me. "What's up?"

"I'm concerned about your health. Jude is getting up about every ninety minutes at night. Which means so are you. I want to find a solution so you can get more sleep."

I felt my body tighten, "I'm doing the best I can, given the circumstances."

Charlie saw me getting defensive, so he made it clear we were on the same team and he was taking care of, not attacking, me. "You're doing great. You're the best mom to Jude, and Jude and I are lucky to have you."

With that, I started to cry, and it was easier to open up about my dilemma. "I really do want more sleep. I'm scared some nights driving home from work that I'll fall asleep at the wheel. But I'm worried that if Jude doesn't drink as much at night, my milk supply won't be enough to nurse him till he's one."

"Why do you think you need to nurse him till he's one, babe?"

"Because that's what Dr. Woods said. I am afraid if I don't, I won't be a good mom."

Charlie said nothing, just leaned in and put his arms around me as I sobbed. I cried for a long time before we talked more.

Finally I said, "Thanks. I needed that cry. I can see I'm giving Dr. Woods insider status. I'm also giving my fears about not being a good-enough mom insider status."

Charlie reassured me that we were the only insiders. He said he understood how much pressure is put on new moms and promised that we'd figure this out together. We began to hatch a plan, asserting our insider status and giving all the advice its appropriate outsider status. After a few more discussions, we arrived at a sleeping decision that worked for our family: transitioning Jude to his own room so he would wake up less often. Working collaboratively as equals helped us navigate the transition with solid footing, which, in turn, helped

Jude. I'll never know for sure, but I believe he could sense his parents' support for each other as well as for him sleeping in his own room, and that made the first couple of nights less challenging for him.

Support from Outside

As parents, you will frequently find yourselves facing decisions for which you have no previous experience to draw from. You two want to make the final decision as a team, but still need an entire support staff of experts, doctors, other parents, friends, family, blog posts, and so on for necessary information. You've never been parents before, and your child is always changing and growing, keeping the learning curve steep. It's not necessary to reinvent the wheel, but it is necessary to decide together which wheel you're rolling with.

Suppose you're unsure about when to wean your child. So you consult a logical outsider: your pediatrician. Your partner is working, so you go alone with your child. The pediatrician suggests this is a good time to wean your child. You listen, and then you conjure up your insider force field and say, "Great, thank you. I'll discuss it with my partner."

When you get home, you don't say, "This is what the pediatrician said, and we're weaning now." You relay the pediatrician's advice and ask for your partner's thoughts. Then you decide together.

Or a friend asks, "What preschool is your daughter going to attend?"

You guys haven't decided yet, so you say, "We're not sure. Which one did you pick?"

When you get home, you tell your partner which preschool your friend has selected, and you two add that info to the decision you're already working on.

Baby as an Outsider

Your status as insiders becomes all the more necessary to practice once baby is here, because baby is an outsider. I know that sounds harsh, but by encouraging your self-care as a team, your insider force field actually protects baby. When you are strong as a team, you can better nurture and protect your child.

For example, when your child gets older and starts hitting up one of you for, say, ice cream instead of fruit, you say no. So your child runs and asks your partner. Now, if you and your partner have a weak team, your child may be able to weasel the treat out of your partner. Then not only are you angry at your child, but you and your partner are angry at each other as well. The next time your child asks for ice cream, it will be harder for either of you to provide a confident no.

On the other hand, if you and your partner are a secure team, your partner will immediately reference what you just said, and it'll be case closed: no ice cream. To be honest, your child may want the treat, but they'd rather have two parents on the same page.

Sometimes you may change a decision based on your child's input as an outsider. Take the ice cream over fruit scenario. Your child asks you for a treat, and you say no and suggest fruit instead. They don't like your answer, so they go to your partner with the request.

Your partner thinks, *They haven't had ice cream all week. I don't think it's a bad idea to allow some now.* Your partner doesn't say this aloud but says, "Let me check on this."

The two of you discuss this in your insider cave, sans child. By listening and talking, you can decide together if your child gets a treat or not.

Using Your Insider Status

The following is a list of some big parenting decisions you will need to make as a couple. Feel free to add to this list or make the items more specific.

- your child's sleep schedule

- your child's nutrition

- your child's education

- your child's activities

- your child's use of screen time

- your child's health care

- discipline for your child

If you are an expecting (or hope-to-be) parent, go through this list with your partner and discuss who your outsiders will be for each decision. Consider which outsiders you want to include and discuss how you will go about engaging with each of them. If you're already parents, name your current or past outsiders or hatch a plan to find some.

Discuss any concerns you have about outsiders who could make it harder for you as insiders. Consider how easily you can be influenced by experts or your own parents when it comes to certain parenting decisions. The more insider info you can gather about how you and your partner will navigate your outsiders' influence, the better. Know which outsiders are the biggest influencers, and continue to grow your outsider village.

What Makes This Principle Hard?

Putting the guiding principle that you and your partner make decisions as a team into practice can be tricky. As we've discussed, the culture around us can make it hard. Some powerful cultural messages are at odds with you two making decisions as a team. Also, if you are already a parent and have a history in your twosome of making decisions as a onesome, it's possible you don't know how to shift gears. Here we look at three areas of difficulty and some tips on how to combat them.

Moms Should Be in Charge

"What kind of stroller did you decide to get?" "How long are you planning to stay home with baby?" "Are you making baby's food from scratch?" "If you're here, then who's with baby?" "You're lucky to have such an involved father!"

The problem here is not the questions themselves or that one partner (unless you're in a lesbian couple) is being complimented. The problem is that these kinds of questions are directed at moms, not dads. To be a great mom in our culture, you must do it all effortlessly and perfectly because you were born to do it; it's your life's true work. This includes making the right decisions at the right time for baby. To be a great dad, you simply have to show up and change a diaper occasionally or take your kid to the park.

This cultural messaging is harmful to all genders. That harm is nowhere more apparent than in the decision-making process. If you as a mom feel it's on you to make all the parenting decisions, you will have half the resources you need to research and choose the best solution. When you read about the team decision-making process I presented, a little voice in your mind will say, *But that's really my responsibility.* You may feel making team decisions is an imposition on your partner or that outsiders will think less of you if you take extra time to make decisions as a team.

This messaging can be especially challenging if you buy into it unconsciously. You may think, *Of course, we want to do this as a team!* At the same time, below the surface, part of your psyche may cause you to feel guilty about going against this message. The same applies to your partner, who also may buy in either consciously or unconsciously.

Same-sex couples tend to struggle less with this specific cultural message. I've noticed many same-sex partners prefer to engage in a continual conversation about roles and responsibilities, rather than adhere to culturally driven assumptions about gender. If you are in a same-sex partnership, you may find this freedom allows you to practice this chapter's guiding principle with greater ease.

How do you counter this messaging? If you're struggling with this message (in a same-sex or opposite-sex partnership), there are ways to counter it. Together with your partner, make it a goal to become acutely aware of the cultural messaging about moms and dads. Over the next week, slow down and notice the different expectations for each gender. Pay attention to advertisements, television shows, conversations at work, social media posts, and articles.

- Which gender is addressed most often when it comes to parenting?

- What are the expectations for your gender? For your partner's gender (if it's different)?

- Notice how you feel about your discoveries.

Increase your awareness individually and then share your findings with your partner. Discuss what each of you noticed and the impact of the messaging on your decision-making.

You Can't Agree on a Decision

Even after trying the process I've given for making decisions as a team, you and your partner may still find yourselves on different sides of the fence. You might be at loggerheads about sleeping arrangements or vehemently disagree about getting pregnant again. It can be especially difficult if a decision was already made before you started this process. For example, baby may have been conceived without mutual agreement, leaving one or both of you with nagging resentments and making it harder to trust your decision-making process going forward.

How do you get on the same page? If you and your partner can't agree on a particular decision, try giving yourselves a little breather and then revisit it. Sometimes the extra time is all it takes for partners to get on the same page. However, if you're dealing with fallout from an earlier decision that can't be reversed, you may benefit from extra support. There is no stigma attached to seeking couple therapy to resolve issues that keep you from functioning as a solid team.

You've Been Making Decisions Separately

If you and your partner are in the habit of making decisions without consulting each other, even if the new model appeals to you, it can be hard to shift over. Or you may try it out, because it sounds good, but then flub up, because you aren't used to making decisions as a team. For example, if one of you has been making all the decisions about babysitters, you may both take that groove for granted. If you're the babysitter czar, you may not trust your partner to vet sitters properly. It may feel easier to keep doing the job solo, even if your resentment over the unequal workload is growing. Or your partner may try to share in these decisions but run aground due to unequal access to the list of sitters you've been working from.

All in all, switching things up so you can make decisions as a team can feel like a boatload of extra work. It may not seem worth the bother. So let me give you some motivation. In the babysitter example, you can reap many benefits when both of you are able to book sitters. First, sharing this responsibility creates more equal parenting. Second, the parent who hasn't booked sitters before has an opportunity to increase parenting self-confidence. Third, taking turns booking sitters can help with self-care. For instance, if you're too pressed for time to find a sitter, you might cancel date night; however, passing that task to your partner might give you enough rest to save your date night. Both of you sharing responsibility for childcare can bring a spirit of appreciation that's absent when it remains a one-person show and that person's behind-the-scenes work is invisible.

How do you shift gears in this situation? The first step is realizing the value of it. You can get clear about this by asking yourself several questions:

- Do I make sure my partner is an insider in all our decisions?

- Have I been as transparent in sharing info with my partner as I'd like to be?

- Do I ever leave my partner on the hook to make decisions alone?

You can also ask how your partner experiences your involvement in decision-making:

- Did you think I was a team player when we shopped for our baby registry?

- I think I could have been more collaborative. What do you think?

- Was I involved in all our decisions when you were pregnant?

You may discover that you've been asleep at the wheel during some big decisions or that you haven't included your partner. Either way, knowing this and owning it is a big step forward.

This next step is seeing how your behavior affects your partner, and vice versa. We'll cover in chapter 9 how to apologize to one another, but for now you can start by having open and supportive conversations. Notice any patterns when you have a lapse in team decision-making. For example, notice if an outsider has been given insider status, or any specific parenting decisions that are harder to collaborate on than others.

Conclusion

From the moment you find out you're expecting, you and your partner enter a new world of decisions to make together. You both deserve each other's help in making these decisions, and you both deserve to have your opinions valued. This process takes practice, kindness, and openness. As secure-functioning co-captains, you can alert each other to each decision as it arises and stay with one another until you make your team decision. Use the concept of insiders and outsiders to strengthen your team and to clarify the role of your extended team. Be aware when things run amuck and work together to get back on track.

In the next chapter, we'll dig into the impact of baby's arrival on your partnership. We'll explore how to get in touch with your own needs once baby is here and how to involve your partner in addressing those needs. We'll also look at how to help your partner with their needs. Valuing each other's needs will keep your team strong and successful.

CHAPTER 5

Reality Hits

Congrats, your baby bomb has hit the scene! Now tell me ... do any of the following moments sound familiar?

You're standing in your kitchen, holding your precious, crying baby bomb. You've watched Dr. Harvey Karp's videos about the 5 S's to soothe your baby and exhausted every single S, and your baby's still wailing away. You're frantic to know what your baby needs so you can provide it, but you have absolutely no clue what it is.

Or ... after much rocking and singing, you successfully help your baby fall asleep. You look over at the door—your exit from parenting and entrance into a much-needed reprieve—and it suddenly feels like that door has leapt twenty feet farther away. You wish you could magically levitate toward it and slip out without making a peep. But even your best ninja moves don't do the trick: your baby hears you, wakes up, and cries. You're back at square one, defeated, and wondering, "How will I ever get you to sleep again?"

Or ... you're driving yourself and your baby to a parenting class. Somehow you've managed to get both of you out the door and are about to be miraculously on time for class. Awesome! But then you smell it: the distinct odor of poop. You think, *Please, not another diaper blowout!* The odor is so strong you're freaked about how much mess must be back there. When you park and pull your baby out of the car seat, you discover poop everywhere—all over your baby, their clothes, the seat. You look up at the sky and whisper, "Help me!" But you know it's on you to figure out how to clean up the whole mess, as well as what you'll do with your baby while you're working on it.

You probably weren't thinking about moments like these when you placed your order for a delicious baby bomb. Of course, there are other moments you couldn't have anticipated in their full richness either, such as staring spellbound at your newborn, wondering how such a fantastic creature could ever exist. Or the moment your baby looks up at you and laughs for the first time— loving you, and you loving your baby right back. You want to freeze-frame the sheer magic. Or the moment you watch your partner climb the Everest of figuring out how to soothe your baby bomb, and you know you've never had more admiration for your partner's patience and attunement.

Becoming parents can open a door within each of you that you didn't know existed. As Tina Fey famously said after becoming a parent, "You go through big chunks of time where you're just thinking, 'This is impossible—oh, this is impossible.' And then you just keep going and keep going, and you sort of do the impossible." You learn to climb each new Everest. If you're reading this and your baby bomb is en route, buckle up and get ready to live the impossible every day. If your baby bomb is already here, you likely know what I'm talking about.

Meeting this new reality is harder if you aren't in right relationship with your needs. The guiding principle in this chapter is about valuing your own and your partner's needs. Identifying and meeting your needs and helping your partner do the same is critical to being successful as parents and partners. This may sound counterintuitive. Why focus on *your* needs when you have a little buddy whose needs must come first and who requires so much of your attention? The mantra of this book is to care for yourself and your partnership *so that* you can best care for your baby.

I've already mentioned the emergency instructions we always hear on planes: put on your own oxygen mask before helping your child. The same is true when it comes to valuing your needs. Putting on the oxygen mask of valuing your own needs allows you to provide a secure base for both your partner and your child. Babies' vulnerability during their first few months of life is intense in its sheer magnitude. They can't even hold up their heads when they're born. They need help eating, burping, sleeping, and bonding. They can't do anything without your help. But to be able to help them—as our metaphor says—you first need to take care of your own needs.

In this chapter, we first look at how to identify your own needs as a new parent. This includes how your needs have shifted with your new parent status. I provide some tools to help you discover or rediscover how to care for yourself. Then we explore how you can continually value your needs and your partner's needs and effectively communicate that value within your family. Bargaining for win-wins with your partner will help you maintain this as a daily practice. We also consider a commonly overlooked need of new parents: the need to feel confident in their ability to parent.

Guiding Principle 5: You and your partner value your own and each other's needs.

Pre-parenthood, it was probably easier to keep your finger on the pulse of your needs. You likely knew you needed sleep, food, love, play, connection, time alone, couple time, exercise, creative time, work time—to name some of the most obvious. Life post-baby has a different feel to it. Your needs may have shifted significantly, with new needs cropping up that you never considered before. You may even feel out of touch with what your needs are. When you're out of touch with them, it's hard to value your needs. I can speak to that myself.

One afternoon during my early postpartum days, having just gotten Jude down for a nap, I walked into our living room, where Charlie was restringing his guitar.

"Hey love, how're you doing?" he asked, putting down the guitar.

"I'm okay," I said. "Jude's asleep. Oh my God, Charlie, he's so adorable while he sleeps. I love watching him sleep, our little bug!"

"Me too. He's so special," Charlie agreed, then looked at me closely. He could see how fatigued I was, just running on adrenaline. "Why don't you do something special for yourself? You haven't left the house without Jude since he was born."

That's when the full force of the baby bomb really hit me. Not only had I not thought of talking to Charlie about leaving the house alone, I had no idea what to do for downtime now that I was a mom. It was a startling and surreal moment. "Honestly," I said, "I don't know what I'd do with myself. I can't touch the part of me that knew myself so well before I was a mom. I'm feeling so vulnerable and lost right now."

Charlie came over and hugged me, and his embrace felt soothing to my nervous system. But I knew what I needed most in that moment was to connect with myself, not with him or anyone else. So I quickly hugged him back, thanked him, and went upstairs. I grabbed a notebook and got down to the business of discovering who I was now, what I needed for myself, and what I might still enjoy doing alone.

At the end of an hour, I had compiled a list of what I used to like to do in my downtime. My list was long, but I decided to focus on my top three: exercise, time with other moms sans babies, and cuddle time with Charlie. Later, he made his own list, which revealed that he wanted time to work on his creative projects, cuddle time with me, and quiet alone time. Together, we hatched a plan whereby we would both step up and step down as parents so our respective needs could be not just checked off on a list but fully valued and met.

The truth of the baby bomb is that both you and your partner have become different people. Paradoxically, while you're still the same in many ways, you are forever changed. There is so much to understand and integrate. It's time to get to know this person you are now and what you like and don't like, need and don't need.

First consider your basic needs—sleep, exercise, work, food, showers, and so on. Although these basic needs remain consistent from pre-parenthood to parenthood, meeting them can become difficult. For example, during pregnancy, your ability to exercise, sleep soundly, and experience sexual desire can be thrown off by body shape and hormone changes. Eating meals can become a daily adventure: will you be making a trip to the bathroom before or after your meal today? Morning sickness can change your relationship to food. When you have a newborn, taking a shower can seem impossible for a while. Then, almost before you realize it, it's part of your routine again.

Next consider your higher needs, which reflect how you want to spend your time on this planet. They may have nothing to do with baby or your partner and instead be activities you do for yourself. Or they may be things you'd like to do with your baby, with your partner, or with both of them. Examples include dancing, going out with friends, hiking, painting, reading, a day at the spa, playing sports, gardening, band practice, surfing, golf, going to religious services, swimming.

When reality hits as a new parent, you may tell yourself these higher needs are out of the picture for the foreseeable future. You may see them as inaccessible aspects of the pre-parent you. You may even feel guilty for entertaining the thought of pursuing them.

I'm here to say that ignoring your higher needs won't work. These needs and desires light you up, recharge your batteries, and give you oxygen. Engaging in them is essential to your ability to be secure functioning and to your well-being as a person, parent, and partner.

Reconnecting with the Pre-Parent You

The purpose of this exercise is to assess your needs as a new parent. Even if you haven't struggled with this as I did, I suggest trying the exercise anyway. You might discover some aspects of yourself you weren't aware of.

To start, you will need a notebook (or digital equivalent) and some undistracted time for yourself. You may want to bring along some tea or coffee or whatever would be a treat for yourself and make this alone time feel special. Ideally, your partner will also want to do this exercise on their own so you can compare notes.

The exercise has two parts: meditation (five minutes) and journaling (twenty-five minutes). The brief meditation is intended to reconnect you with your body before you begin to reconnect with yourself on a mental-emotional level.

Meditation

1. Sit in a comfortable position, with your hands on your knees or in your lap, and close your eyes.

2. Notice your breath, paying attention to the inhale and exhale, without changing anything.

3. Now bring your attention to your hands; notice them. Ask yourself: *Can I feel my hands? Can I feel the air touching my hands?*

4. See what happens as you continue to bring your awareness to your hands. Do they feel warm or tingly? It may be helpful to gently rub them back and forth to experience the sensations and reconnect with your body.

5. Bring your attention back to your breath and notice your body breathing itself. Open your eyes.

Journaling

1. Make a list of all the things you loved to do before becoming a parent. Try not to censor yourself. The goal is to get an idea of who you were and how you liked to spend your time.

2. Pick three things from this list you could bring into your life now.

3. Take your list to your partner. If both of you have done this exercise, you can figure out together how to incorporate your respective three things into

your lives on a regular basis. If your partner doesn't participate in this exercise, don't let that stop you from finding ways to make time for yourself.

4. Keep adding to your list over the coming days and weeks. Allow yourself to be surprised: you may recall more things or discover new ones. Keep the list handy so when you stumble into some free time, you can easily find a way to nourish yourself.

Valuing Each Other's Needs

So you've begun to value your needs by taking the time to identify them and incorporate them into your life, but in a secure-functioning relationship, there's another side to the act of valuing. Valuing must be consistently communicated between you and your partner. Consider how this works—or doesn't—for Greta and Peter.

Greta is getting two-year-old Sophie ready for bed. Her teeth are brushed, her jammies on, and it's time to read a book before tucking her in. A quick glance at the clock tells Greta she's late to meet her buds, Erica and Camila, for drinks. "Pete!" she calls out, loud enough for him to hear over the television blaring in the living room.

A minute later, Peter pops his head in. "Ready for bed?" he asks.

"Almost," Greta says. "If you'll just read to Sophie …."

But Sophie already has a book in hand and a clear idea about how this should go. "Mommy read!" she cries. "Mommy read!"

"Mommy can't read," Peter scoffs. Greta told him at dinner she was going out, but he assumed she'd handle bedtime first, giving him time to watch the game.

"*Of course* I can read," Greta says, as if her literacy skills are in question. "I'll do it tomorrow."

"Mommy read!" Sophie wails.

Peter shoots Greta a "see what you've done" look and hisses, "Just go!"

"I'll be back by nine at the latest, babe." Greta plants a kiss on Sophie's head, then slips out. *He always sabotages things I want to do for myself,* she thinks. *I do so much around the house. I deserve some open-ended time off the mom clock!*

Peter picks up Sophie and is about to read to her, but she's fussing too much. Suddenly he has an idea—a treat for Sophie that could work for both of them. "Hey kiddo, how about watching TV with Daddy?"

That does the trick. Sophie stops crying and dashes toward the living room, landing on the couch before Peter can get there. Pleased with himself, he tucks her in with the afghan throw so they can be cozy together. He gets so relaxed watching his team coast to a win that he's fast asleep before the game ends.

Next thing he knows, Sophie is awake and crying, and it's after midnight. As he tries to soothe her, he turns off the television and reaches for his phone to check messages. *Where is Greta?* he fumes. He manages to get Sophie quiet and into bed, and sits by her until she is asleep.

Just as he finally returns to the living room, Greta walks in. He greets her with anger: "It's after midnight! You said you'd be back by nine."

"I knew you'd be pissed, so I waited until you'd be asleep," she counters.

"Sophie woke me up. Guess your sneaking around didn't work."

"If you'd let me hang with my friends more, I wouldn't have to sneak around."

Peter knows they should talk about this rationally in the light of day, but he can't let Greta's dig stand. "So it's my fault you got caught? News flash: I'm not your keeper!"

"No, you're not. But I did think you were my *partner.*"

Peter can see from Greta's clenched jaw how crushed she feels, so he softens a tad. "Look, I've got an early meeting. I'm sleeping in the bed, with earplugs in. You can take the baby monitor and sleep on the couch. We'll talk more tomorrow."

As they try to fall asleep, both Peter and Greta wonder how things got so far off track. Peter wonders why she would sneak around, and Greta wonders why he made her sleep on the couch with the baby monitor. Neither of them gets much sleep.

♥♥♥

Peter and Greta seem to have some sense of their individual needs. Greta values time with friends. He values his sports time. For our purposes here, let's assume they have started making lists of their needs. This scenario shows the limited usefulness of such lists in the absence of partners' ability to communicate about their needs. Instead of voicing her needs and negotiating with Peter, Greta feels she has to sneak around. Peter is doing his own sneaking with the television. If that weren't bad enough, their toddler is caught in the friction, her need for love and security taking a back seat while her parents struggle to get their own needs met.

Hashing Out Your Needs Together

Valuing is a two-way street. It's hard to value your partner's needs if they don't value yours. Moreover, it's hard to ask your partner to value your needs if you don't value them yourself. All that is triply hard if you can't talk openly and honestly with each other about these needs. The following are three interlocking practices to make your communication around needs successful.

Self-assess how you value your needs. Constructive communication necessitates that you know and keep track of what you bring to the table. This means checking in with yourself on a continual basis—both before you sit down with your partner and between the times you do. Here are some quick questions to ask yourself a couple times a week.

- What are my needs right now? Think body, mind, and spirit needs.

- Am I actively trying to get my needs met? If so, how is getting them met benefiting me? If not, why not?

- Is my partner helping me get my needs met? If so, how does that feel? If not, how might we change that?

Check in with each other. Each week, get together with your partner and share how successful you each feel you've been with respect to valuing and acting on your respective needs. This includes discussing how supportive each of you feels the other has been, as well as ways you can increase your teamwork. Take turns putting your needs on the table, and use these check-ins to build trust and transparency with each other. As you communicate, use your sherlocking skills: watch your partner's expressions and gestures to detect any clues about what your partner feels about how their needs are getting met.

Negotiate win-wins. It's easy to value and support each other's needs when those needs fit into your lives effortlessly. For example, your partner wants to meditate first thing in the morning before anyone is awake. Or you want to go to the gym after you drop off your son at daycare. In these scenarios, you and your partner can meet your needs without any real negotiation. But what to do when meeting your need requires your partner's help, when it necessitates a joint resolution? In those cases, you and your partner need to find a win-win. We'll cover more about win-wins in chapter 9, but for now, think of win-wins as solutions in which both partners get what they need.

Consider how Peter and Greta could achieve a win-win. If Greta wants a night out without a curfew, she has to coordinate with Peter so his needs aren't left in the lurch. And if Peter wants to watch more sports, he has to bring that need to the table when talking with Greta. In fact, let's give the two of them a chance for a do-over.

Revisiting Peter and Greta

This time, having worked everything out with Peter at dinner, Greta feels at ease as she playfully gives Sophie a bath. "This super washcloth is gonna wash this super girl!"

Sophie giggles. "I'm super girl!"

Just then Peter walks in and says, "Super mama, super girl ... and here's super dad!" They all laugh as he turns to Greta. "I'm ready to take over. You said you have to leave by seven, right?"

"Yep, thanks. I'm super excited to see Erica and Camila."

"We're really embracing this whole *super* thing, huh?" Peter says, laughing.

"Super embracing it," Greta says, then adds, "I didn't ask you earlier, but I'd like to stay out late. Maybe after midnight. Is that okay?"

"Shoot, babe!" Peter frowns. He didn't see that coming. But then he remembers how well they communicated earlier and decides to build on that. "Thing is, I have an early meeting, and I won't sleep well till you're home. Could you do a late night some other time?"

"Aw, I was really feeling it tonight." Greta stops herself when she notices the worry lines deepening on Peter's brow. "But, okay, I get it. What time do you have in mind?"

"How about by ten? Can you work with that, wild woman?"

"I can. And let's look at our calendars so I can plan another night out with the ladies, sans curfew. Deal?"

"Sounds great. Speaking of wanting things ...." Sophie starts to splash in the bath, signaling a timer on her parents' negotiations. Peter grabs some bath toys from the sink and hands them to her to buy a few more minutes. "I miss watching football in real time. I want that in my life again."

"Absolutely. I'm so glad you told me. Maybe I can take Sophie out, and you can have the guys over to watch the game this weekend?"

"Maybe. Let's look at our calendars when you get home and see if we can make plans that work for both of us. But I don't want you to be late now. Kiss Sophie goodbye."

♥♥♥

The biggest change in this scenario is how direct Greta and Peter are about what they want. They pay attention to each other's tells in the moment and take care of each other. Both take stock of what they need and value, and both are committed to working together to figure out how to make that happen. Their negotiation of a win-win looks promising, and I'd be surprised if Greta doesn't get her night out and Peter doesn't get his sports in. Also, Sophie wins from watching how well her parents take care of each other's needs as well as hers.

Feeling Confident as Parents

As Charlie and I were working to value our individual needs as new parents, we got in touch with a whole new set of needs. Specifically, we needed to know we could successfully care for Jude and ourselves. We discovered this in the midst of a really challenging experience.

One night, I was holding Jude, and he was crying. As I rocked him back and forth while he wailed, I called out to Charlie, "I don't know what he wants! I've offered him my breast. I've swaddled and re-swaddled him. I'm doing that thing he likes—when I lift him high and swing him down low—but nothing is working. I feel like a total failure!" With that, I started to cry, giving Jude a run for his money.

Charlie came over and lifted my head up so I could see his face and said, "You're doing great. You're a fantastic mom. Jude is so lucky to have you. Let me give it a go, and you take a break."

I handed him to Charlie and gratefully walked away from the crying scene. I could feel my whole body relax. Charlie's words rang in my ears. I thought, *I am a good mom. I wasn't able to figure out what Jude needed, and I'm still a good mom.* I kept repeating this to myself until I started to feel better in my own skin.

When the feeling of failure had left me, I walked back to the crying scene (Jude hadn't relented) and said, "Can I hold him again? I want to give it another go. I'm not feeling desperate anymore."

Jude kept crying. I held him close and started to sing Janis Joplin's "Me and Bobby McGee." As I sang, I almost forgot Jude was inconsolable. I became lost in my role of mother—the role I felt I couldn't live up to ten minutes before. The only thing that had changed was that I believed in myself now.

Confidence in parenting doesn't automatically arrive with baby. It comes from experience and support. The tricky part is that baby can't say, "You're doing a great job, Mom. Thank you!" Or "I see you're trying to help me, Dad. Let me give you a hint—I have diaper rash. That's why I'm fussy." None of that happens in early parenthood. Instead, it's a lot of fumbling around in the dark, manically searching the internet for answers, and endless experimenting on what baby could want now. You're learning a whole new skill set (caring for baby) but not receiving much direct feedback from your boss (baby). It can be a challenging endeavor, for sure.

Charlie and I discovered that helping each other build confidence as parents was a need we didn't even realize we had. As we worked to gain our footing in this new world, Jude was not going to be our go-to cheerleader; he was busy being a baby. We had to do it for ourselves. I've chosen to highlight the need for confidence in this chapter because I think it's easy for new parents to focus on more commonly recognized needs and overlook this important one.

Take an example from the beginning of the chapter. Your baby has a diaper blowout at an inopportune moment, and you're overwhelmed by the prospect of cleaning it up. Who else in this world can understand not only how much you love your baby but also how frazzled you are? Your partner can! Your partner can empathize with your concern about doing a good job and provide the reassurance you need. And you can do this for your partner.

Your mutual vulnerability as new parents becomes your point of connection and salvation during stressful moments. The flip side applies as well: if neither of you recognizes how vulnerable you are and tends to the other's vulnerabilities, these moments can tear you down. Supporting each other's development as parents is a foundational step to meeting your many other partnering and parenting needs. The more confident you feel as a parent, the more you'll jump in and parent so your partner can get their needs met, and vice versa. You become expert cheerleaders for each other. Here are two cheerleading tips to help you build parenting confidence.

Provide your partner with frequent positive feedback. As I mentioned, your baby won't be providing articulate feedback. You'll have to do it. Often. Noticing each other's attempts and being generous in your compliments can provide the boost in confidence that makes all the difference. There is no downside to saying (and saying often), "I think you're a great dad!" or "You're the best mom!"

Be sensitive when offering corrective feedback. When things are clearly not working, and you want to provide constructive feedback, try the sandwich technique. The format is simple: (1) you start by complimenting a strength, (2) you add a suggestion for something to work on, and (3) you finish with another strength. In my home, this might look like this: "I love how you play with Jude. You're so present and silly. I think when you offer him five food options at dinnertime, he may feel overwhelmed and unable to choose. I think he's too young for that. I love how you make mealtime fun by playing airplane when you're feeding him. You're such a great dad."

An alternative to the sandwich technique is to ask your partner what they think. For example, I could say to Charlie, "I think we're offering Jude too many options at dinner; I'm not sure he's developmentally ready for that. What do you think?"

Parents are born when their first baby is born, but it can take time to build confidence as a parent. That starts with recognizing and valuing your need for confidence. We generally pull away from doing things when we feel we're not good at them. So building confidence will help you both become more involved as parents.

What Makes This Principle Hard?

Valuing your own needs and your partner's needs as parents can be a delicate, often challenging, balancing act. The mainstream culture's focus on nuclear family isolation doesn't encourage parents to value their own needs. Another obstacle is on the personal level: your and your partner's attachment colors can get in the way of valuing your needs. Let's look at these two issues more closely and consider ways to combat them.

Culture Doesn't Support Valuing Needs

"We'd love to be there, but we don't have childcare." "A date night would be fun, but we can't afford a sitter." "The day-care center waitlist is months long. I don't know what we'll do in the meantime."

In many modern-day families, most of the responsibility for raising children rests on two people—the parents—without supporting cast members to lend a hand, do a drop-off, or jump in at a moment's notice. "It takes a village" is common wisdom, but that village is absent for too many families these days. Moreover, many parents are part of a "sandwich generation," taking care of their parents at the same time that they are new parents themselves. It's hard to fill up your own cups, as parents, when the culture is constantly conveying the message that anything that doesn't prioritize your child's or your own parents' cups is self-indulgence.

This plays out in the larger community in the form of lack of low-cost childcare, maternity and paternity leave, and other support systems that would help parents find the space to tend to their own needs. Instead, in this country, most are forced to carry the burdens of parenting alone. This is a systemic problem and not something you and your partner can fix on your own. However, you may want to consider getting more involved in activism that supports these policy changes.

What else can you do about it? For starters, you can build your own village—that is, your support system for emotional and logistical help. Unless you have extended family nearby, you will need to think in terms of a friend network. Building a village may sound daunting, but it's easier than you think. Also, you may be surprised by how grateful your new village is that you initiated the connection.

Here are some ideas for locating your village. Basically, any place where kids hang out probably has super cool parents like you who are also hungry for connection and support.

- daycare or preschool

- parks

- indoor play spaces

- zoos and museums

- your neighborhood

- social media parenting groups

Once you've met some peeps and collected phone numbers or email addies, it's time to put them to work. Schedule play hangs with your kids as well as get-togethers minus kiddos. Kids' playdates help their relationships, but you may only have a few minutes of adult time before an interruption. The get-togethers minus the kiddos allow for the longer conversation necessary to create friend-ships, and they give you opportunities to bring your respective partners into the mix. It takes time to develop relationships, so don't be deterred if you feel new-friend awkwardness for a while. And don't rush into shared childcare. Each relationship in your village will be unique: some may naturally evolve into prac-tical support, while others may be more about fulfilling purely social needs. Once you've built your village, use it however you can—whether that looks like childcare for a night on the town, a playdate, or something else.

Attachment Colors Obscure Needs

Learning to value our needs and self-worth can be a lifelong practice. In particular, those who hang out in the blue and red parts of the attachment continuum may find this practice especially challenging. People with blue and red styles typically didn't have their needs consistently valued and met as chil-dren, which can lead them to feel shame about having needs as an adult or even to deny their needs altogether. This can show up in your partnership in a variety of ways. For example, like Peter and Greta in the first version of their scenario, you may struggle to directly name what you need, or you may sneak around to get your needs met without your partner's help or involvement.

If this is you, try not to sweat it too much. Just knowing this is a challenge for you is half the battle. When you become aware of an inner struggle, it begins to lose some of its hold on you. To do this, claim some uninterrupted quiet time to journal about your relationship with needs. Consider these questions:

- How were my needs valued as a child?

- Did anyone help me get my higher-level needs met? If so, how did that feel? If not, how is that lack of support affecting me now?

- How do I want my child(ren) to feel about having needs?

I mention the last point because your child is watching how you and your partner value your own needs. Your young one is collecting data on what it means to be an adult. Seeing you care for yourself will make your child more likely to believe their needs also deserve to be met—now and as an adult.

You may find it painful to look back at your childhood. Delving into the past can bring up attachment wounding—that is, it can remind you of ways you felt hurt by your caregivers when you were young and vulnerable. So be gentle with yourself. And take the help of your partner. Sit down together and discuss how your attachment colors might be affecting your ability to value your own needs and to ask directly for them to be met.

Conclusion

Now that your baby bomb is here, it's time to initiate a new lifelong personal and relational conversation about needs. You, your partner, and your baby bomb are in it for the long game, so how you choose to fulfill your needs has to work for all three of you. This means you and your partner have to identify and support each of your needs in an equal and balanced manner. In this chapter, we covered how to reconnect with your basic needs, as well as your higher-level needs, including the need to feel confident as a parent.

One need we haven't talked explicitly about is the need to rejuvenate yourselves now that you've become a party of three. In the next chapter, we'll expand on what you learned in chapter 2 about becoming experts on each other. I'll show you how to apply those skills (and more) for the much-needed purpose of relationship restoration.

CHAPTER 6

Relationship Restoration

Having refused both his naps today, Ezra is fussy on his blanket in the living room. His chubby fingers lift up a toy only to petulantly throw it back down. Due to his son's nap strike, Dylan hasn't been able to do any of the things he planned for naptime: return emails, wash dishes, meal prep, even a quick workout. These aren't glamorous things, but they give Dylan a sense of calm and order. Now, instead, he feels tired, irritated, and impatient to see his wife, Cassie.

He scoops up Ezra and tries to soothe him by walking around the living room. "Mama will be here soon," he croons. "She knows the trick to get you to sleep. We just have to make it till she walks through that door." *Which better be soon!* he thinks.

Meanwhile, Cassie is irritated and frazzled herself. Work was especially grueling, with a meeting that ran late. Which means rush hour was in full swing by the time she reached the freeway. She taps the steering wheel repeatedly as she gazes at the sea of brake lights and realizes her normal half-hour commute will be over an hour. She'd better let Dylan know. So she dials his number. When he doesn't pick up, she leaves a voicemail. "Babe, I'm going to miss dinner. Please don't wait for me. I'm sorry."

As soon as she has hung up, her phone rings. It's Dylan. "Where *are* you?" he asks, without saying hello.

"Stuck in traffic. My meeting …"

"You're still on the freeway?" Dylan sounds horrified.

"Didn't you get my voicemail?"

"No. I've had my hands full all day with Ezra. Speaking of which, he's pulling on the dog again. Gotta go!"

It's dark when Cassie finally arrives home. As she walks through the front door, she can hear crying. She hurries into the living room, where Dylan is trying to quiet a famished Ezra. "What the …?" she exclaims. "I told you to feed him and not wait for me."

"And I told you I didn't listen to your voicemail. I haven't been able to do anything I wanted today." Dylan sounds fatigued and frustrated.

Cassie sighs. "I don't know why I bother to leave voicemails if you never listen to them."

Dylan immediately feels defensive. "Ezra hasn't napped all day, and I'm coming unglued—and you walk in an hour late and yell at me for not listening to a *voicemail?* That's not fair, Cassie."

But Cassie is angry too. "Life's not fair. I've been in traffic for the last ninety minutes. I had to pump in the car, and my day was awful too. Being home with Ezra, nap or no nap, would be better than the day I had." With that, she takes Ezra to the kitchen to feed him.

Dylan starts to follow her so he can throw together some dinner. But he's afraid they'll just keep arguing about whose day was worse. *I'm not hungry anyway,* he tells himself as he goes outside and sits on the porch alone. His heart sinks, and he starts to tear up.

♥♥♥

Life can be so wild with baby here. And by "wild," I mean wild. The highs are so high, and the lows can be super low. Like Cassie and Dylan, you're bouncing from red to blue on the attachment continuum, not to mention zip-lining on the nervous system continuum. It's easy to become overwhelmed by caring for your baby, by work, by traffic, and by any and all of life's myriad stressors. In the last chapter, I advised you to value each other's needs—but you may find all that going out the window as the stress piles on. The solution is to value and attend to one often-overlooked need: ample relationship-restoration time. Restoration doesn't just have to be limited to a date night away from baby (though those can provide fun connection time); there are many ways to help each other's nervous systems equalize and to metabolize life stress, without leaving home.

In this chapter, we deepen your and your partner's skill set to care for each other using rituals designed for calm connection during busy days with baby. These rituals can be integrated into your life to bring ease and loving contact, not more work. The guiding principle of coregulation builds on what you learned in chapter 2 about nervous system regulation, sherlocking, and the ability to soothe or excite your partner.

Guiding Principle 6: You and your partner coregulate.

I often think of the Talking Heads song "This Must Be the Place" when I contemplate coregulation. It describes two people completely in sync, such that neither can tell who's leading and who's following. It's a fluid and lightning-fast dance of back and forth, back and forth. This kind of dance can provide the restoration partners need. As you learn to coregulate, you'll build a repertoire of restorative dance moves that will be there for you when you need them most.

This guiding principle operates on both a macro (attachment theory) and a micro (nervous system) level. First we'll explore what you and your partner can do to coregulate at the macro level by strengthening and maintaining your attachment bond with each other. Then we'll delve into the micro level and see in more minute detail how you can use nervous-system regulation to keep your dance going.

In *Wired for Love*, Stan suggests that couples use times of transition— waking up, going to sleep, separations, and reunions—as a starting point for practicing coregulation. Such transitions can test the durability of partners' attachment to each other. It's easy to see how transitions are disruptive for children. For example, your child may feel secure in your love at home, but when you go out—even briefly—your child needs extra reassurance to develop trust that mommy or daddy will return. Even moving away from play and toward a diaper change can go more smoothly if you give extra attention to that transition.

Adults aren't so different. We never fully outgrow the challenge of transitions. Exiting one activity and entering another is a time of heightened stress. This stress can be obvious, such as saying goodbye to your partner at the airport, knowing you'll be apart for a week. Or it can be subtler, such as going to sleep at night. You might think going to sleep happens daily, so no problem, right? Not really. Sleep is the closest we come to death in daily life, and our psyche knows that. The same goes for leaving the dream world and returning to the waking world. These are vulnerable times because we can never be 100 percent certain the separation won't be permanent. And that reality is scary.

When you're still a party of two, it's not hard to build in restoration time as you face transitions and other stressors. For example, you can connect on the horn at any hour, without worrying about childcare. And there's always

Saturday morning in bed, which can last past noon. Or if one of you has to go out of town for business, it might not be a stretch to occasionally arrange for the other to go along. In a secure-functioning twosome, you learn to use these times to nourish connection and intimacy. But now, as a party of three, if you try to imagine finding easy times for restoration, you probably feel like all bets are off.

Coregulation Rituals

In fact, all bets are not off. Restoration time is equally as important, if not more so, in your party of three—you just have to learn innovative ways to create it. An opportunity occurs each time you and your partner leave and come home. Stan talks about these times as "launchings" and "landings" you can use to care for your attachment and nervous system needs. You can do this by ritualizing these daily experiences.

You probably already do some launching and landing rituals with your baby or young child. When you leave home, you bend down to your child's level and say that you love them and that you'll be back. The same goes when you come home: you hurry to embrace your child, communicating that they're loved. I think partners who are parents have an advantage over partners in a twosome, because we're already doing these rituals naturally as we build attachment bonds with our children. So it's just a matter of adapting the same kind of care for our partner.

For example, I like to make eye contact with Charlie and wish him well before he leaves, always adding how much I love him. I think of that launching ritual as a magic bullet for a better day. Charlie does the same for me, usually speaking for Jude as well, while Jude's busy being a toddler. I always feel better leaving when I know I'll be missed.

You can use the landing ritual Stan introduced in *Wired for Love*, which he calls the Welcome Home Ritual: partners welcome each other home with a long hug until their bodies are relaxed and restored. Feel free to adapt this for your situation. For example, in a pandemic world, you might welcome each other with sustained eye contact before washing up. Or if you both work at home, your landing ritual can be a hug when you emerge from different rooms in your house. Consider how Cassie and Dylan use their version of a welcome home ritual in this do-over.

Revisiting Cassie and Dylan

When Cassie hits traffic at its peak, her entire body feels the stress. Crawling down the freeway, she busts out her breast pump to tend to her engorged breasts. *Motherhood is a continual exercise in humility,* she thinks as she covers herself with a scarf and situates the pump. Then she auto-dials Dylan to apologize for being late.

"Babe," she says when he doesn't pick up, "if I'm getting voicemail, that must mean your day is as hectic as mine. You know I'll be home as soon as I can. Can't wait to see you!"

Meanwhile, Dylan is bouncing Ezra in a futile effort to soothe him, counting the minutes before Cassie gets home. Glancing at his phone, he sees a missed call and voicemail. His heart drops, intuiting that she's running late. He takes some deep breaths before calling her back.

"I'm so sorry," Cassie says. "My meeting wouldn't end, and now I'm pumping in the effing car."

"Oh, that's rough, luv!"

"How are things there?"

"Not great, and I can't talk now. Ezra didn't nap at all. But I'm excited to see you. Drive safely, and we're ready to love on you when you get here."

An hour later, Dylan hears Cassie's key in the door. He scoops up Ezra and walks over to welcome her. With one arm around Cassie and the other holding Ezra, he hugs her tightly, feeling his own body relax as they embrace.

Cassie pulls back after a few seconds to make eye contact and read Dylan. Seeing the love on his face, she can feel her body begin to relax.

Ezra gives a little giggle.

"I swear," says Dylan, "that's his first happy sound all day." As Cassie reinitiates their hug, he can feel her body alongside his, both sinking into a state of relaxation. Ezra begins to fuss. "That's it, buddy," Dylan says. "Show your mom what it's been like for me today."

Cassie smiles. "Let me give it a go." She takes Ezra and cuddles him, then looks back at Dylan. "Has he …?"

Dylan anticipates what she's about to say. "When I knew you'd be late, I gave him a bottle. But I haven't done anything about dinner yet. I'll bet you're starved."

"No worries," she says, eyes twinkling as she bounces Ezra on her arm. "Our little man can't thank you verbally, but I know he appreciates how you took care of him all day. I sure do. Why don't you take a little well-earned downtime while I throw something together?"

"Are you sure?"

"You know I'd tell you if I wasn't. Now, go!" she says, giving him a playful shove.

Dylan tears up. "Thanks, luv."

♥♥♥

Here, Dylan and Cassie have all the same stressors, yet their experience could hardly be more different. Even in the midst of traffic and a nap strike, they anticipate their reunion. Just knowing they will be there for each other has a calming effect. Their landing ritual—giving each other a welcome-home hug—serves as a concrete expression of their attachment bond, drawing them into secure yellow and solidifying their partner team. Hugging and looking into each other's eyes also works on a physical level, relaxing their nervous systems.

HELLO AND GOODBYE

In this exercise, you and your partner will create coregulatory rituals as a team and experiment with how you'd like to be sent out into the world and welcomed home. Note that this works both for restoration when you've been under stress and also as a preventive measure to fortify you as a unit against the daily onslaught of stress.

1. Pick a week to experiment. Of course, you don't have to stop after a week, but it's helpful to have a timeframe to assess how the ritual works for you.

2. Design the ritual(s) you will use. You can have the same ritual for your hello and your goodbye, or they can differ. Ritual elements to consider include kisses, hugs, eye contact, I love yous, fist bumps, and gentle touches. Discuss ahead of time where your baby or child will be when you launch and land. Keep your ritual to one or two minutes, so they won't feel left out. A short ritual will also minimize the chances of being interrupted or derailed by an emergency, such as a diaper blowout or screaming child. If that does happen, do your ritual as soon after as you can.

3. Take turns. If both of you work outside the home, the person home first should launch or greet the other. If one of you is a stay-at-home parent, take turns being on the receiving and greeting ends.

As you practice over the course of a week, notice how caring for each other's attachment and nervous system needs affects you. Do you feel restored? On an emotional level? On a physical level? Note what works well and what you want to change going forward.

Good Morning and Good Night

This coregulatory ritual can help you and your partner feel loved and connected throughout the day. A morning ritual lets you get out of bed on the right side, so to speak; an evening ritual restores you at the end of the day. You're in this together, so make sure your partner is on board, and do some preplanning together. Consider how each ritual can work best, based on everyone's sleep schedules, including your child's.

1. Pick a week when you're both in town and everyone is healthy. A sick child or partner can add an unneeded obstacle during this experimental phase. Once the ritual is part of your routine, that won't matter.

2. Discuss how you'd both like to be greeted into the day. This can be as simple as a kiss or hug before you roll over and look at your phone. If you both wake around the same time, acknowledge each other before doing anything else. If it's baby waking you, and you have to jump out of bed, your ritual could be just a whispered "I love you." If one of you gets up earlier, you don't have to wake the other; the ritual could be kissing your sleeping partner's forehead. If you have to leave before your partner is up, and if you have time, you could leave a love note in the bathroom.

3. Discuss how to close out the day together. This could be naming something you're grateful for, quietly touching noses, a forehead rub, reading a story, or hugs. Anything goes as long as it helps soothe you to sleep. It doesn't matter who goes to bed first or if you go to bed at the same time. For example, if you're a night owl, visit your partner in bed for the ritual, before returning to your night-owl business.

Notice at the end of the week how your rituals worked. Do you feel a more secure attachment with your partner? Did you sleep better or feel better during the day? Did nothing change? Would you like to adjust your ritual? Share your observations with your partner.

Coregulation at the Micro Level

The coregulation rituals we just talked about not only increase your secure functioning but also have an effect at the level of your nervous system. Whether you're hugging to welcome your partner home, waking your partner up with a kiss, or reading your partner a bedtime story, you are attuning and soothing both of your nervous systems. In fact, the truth is that you don't need a specific ritual: you and your partner can coregulate during just about any activity— while making love or sharing a laugh or cooking dinner or talking about your weekend plans. What brings coregulation into that activity is your awareness at a micro level of what's happening in real time to your respective nervous systems.

In chapter 2, you and your partner played the coregulation game, in which you experimented with moving each other along the nervous-system continuum. In particular, you used sherlocking to identify nonverbal cues and then practiced ways to soothe each other. We're going to expand upon that here so you can integrate the coregulation game into more moments of your day for restoration and connection.

It can help to understand this from a neurobiological perspective. When partners initially fall in love, their nervous systems buzz with excitement when they're physically close. We know from biological anthropologist Helen Fisher that this buzz is created by the neurotransmitters dopamine and norepinephrine, which drive romantic attraction, as well as the androgens and estrogens that drive sexual attraction. When this neuro-cocktail starts to brew, you can't get enough of each other!

But as your relationship moves past the honeymoon phase, and as you begin to focus more on the daily grind of life—which, sooner or later, can include parenting—the novelty and excitement dim. Your brain is busy processing all the incoming data and automating whatever and wherever it can. Of course, this is helpful for many functions. Imagine if every time you went to work, your brain registered your job duties as a novel experience. Or if every time you breastfed your baby, you couldn't rely on your brain's ability to automate. However, the tendency to automate isn't necessarily helpful for romance.

The good news is that you can restore and deepen your connection through intentional coregulation, by using the exercise I call the "coregulation station." It's important to note that this exercise isn't meant to achieve perfect symbiosis with your partner. Rather, it's about fine-tuning your awareness of each other. You may notice yourself coming in and out of awareness as your thoughts steal you from the present moment. When this happens, use your sherlocking skills to bring yourself back. Your partner's tells may be familiar, but the coregulation station invites you to rediscover your partner in a new light. Paradoxically, you can find a place of quiet love and safety, while becoming entranced with a novel experience of each other.

COREGULATION STATION

This is meant to be a meditative experience, with your partner's face as the object of your attention. All you need is time without distraction, the ability to be face to face, and a timer. I suggest a time when baby is asleep for your first experience.

1. Sit close, facing your partner, with your knees touching or close—not more than two feet from each other. It's critical that you both are distraction free. No phones or baby monitors.

2. Set your timer for five minutes, then buckle up for the magic.

3. Gaze at each other, as you sit quietly, without speaking or reaching out. Focus on your partner's face as the object of your attention and study. Notice your partner's eyes, cheeks, lips, nose. Be curious. Notice what it feels like to be seen so deeply by your partner. You may feel nervous at first. That's okay. Just steady yourself with your partner's eyes, and relax your muscles whenever tension arises.

4. When the timer goes off, give each other a silent acknowledgment as you transition out of the experience. This could simply be a smile or reaching out for each other's hands.

5. Discuss your experience of the coregulation station. For example:

   • What did you notice happening in your nervous system? Was the experience calming, exciting, or both?

   • What did it feel like to be gazed at by your partner?

   • Did you learn anything? About yourself? About your partner?

   • Do you feel different as a couple after this exercise?

This exercise can last as long or as short as you wish. Initially gazing for five minutes allows you to settle into coregulation together, and using a timer provides some containment. But feel free to extend the time or forgo the timer, based on your and your partner's nervous systems and attachment needs.

Once you are familiar with it, you can return to the coregulation station whenever you wish and integrate it into your daily life, including times when baby is present. In fact, it's great for your child to see you guys care for each other in this intimate way.

Date Night In

Going on a date night is one obvious way partners seek to bring restoration into their lives. However, it's a big ask for new parents to coordinate regular date nights. You have to contend with childcare, which usually adds to the cost of going out. Especially if you're already physically depleted, just the thought of negotiating the arrangements can be exhausting. Not to mention that external forces—ranging from inclement weather to a global pandemic—can put a damper on your options.

Enter date nights in! I got this idea from some friends, KK and Joseph, whose son is Jude's age. Their faces lit up as they described how they put their son to bed and tidy up their home for date night. Joseph loves to cook, so he prepares a special meal for after baby's bedtime. KK hangs in the kitchen as he cooks, and they listen to music and chat—casual pre-baby style. At first, they made a rule not to talk about their son during date night in, but as it became a weekly event, they decided to discuss him as long as the focus remains on them as partners and parents.

Charlie and I committed to our own weekly date night in. After we turn off electronically, we tune in to each other, using the coregulation station exercise for about ten to fifteen minutes. Having set the tone, we do a variety of things together. Sometimes we cook, sometimes we order in, sometimes we talk, sometimes we cuddle and watch a movie. Some nights include sexual intimacy, others don't. We don't have a rule one way or another. I know couples who plan intimate time as part of each date night in, and that works well for them.

What makes date night in special for Charlie and me is that we're available only to each other and dedicate the time to being restorative and playful together. We don't tackle family planning or troubleshoot problems. On these dates, life feels more like it did pre-Jude. Sometimes I get bored when I can't pick up my phone and engage with it, but Charlie and I discovered that boredom can, in fact, lead us to novelty in the form of new conversations and experiments.

As you and your partner create your own date nights in, here are some things to consider:

- What conversation topics bring us closer?

- Are any topics taboo?

- Do we want to include sex in our date night in?

- Phones and other devices: on or off?

- Does the date night in last all night?

- What happens if, or when, we get bored?

- Who's in charge of dinner? Do we alternate?

- How do we reschedule a date night in that was cancelled due to sickness, fatigue, or anything else?

- What do we miss doing together that we could do during date night in?

- What do we definitely want to keep out of date night in?

Date Night Out

As much fun as date night in can be, there's nothing like being out and about with your partner sans baby. If you can swing childcare and feel rested and adventurous enough, going out with your lover can be a blast.

I like relationship expert Esther Perel's suggestion for daytime dates for new parents, because you'll be more rested, and because childcare can be easier to line up, especially during the day on weekends. I also like her "nights out without a curfew" if family or friends can take baby for the night. Knowing you don't have to rush home for the sitter can fire up your night. I know one couple who surprised themselves by bowling for hours on a night without a curfew, and another who spontaneously went to a bar with a live band and danced for the first time in ages.

What if your family lives too far away? Or you're shy about asking friends? Time to build your village! Friends of ours, Sarah and Darío, have a boy about Jude's age. After bonding over wild parenting experiences, we offered to help each other with date nights (the kind *with* a curfew), but it took at least a year of friendship and playdates before we took the plunge. Now I go over to their house and hang with their son, put him to bed, and watch television until they come home. Darío is usually the one who does it for us. I'd love to find more families to share in this way.

As you and your partner plan date nights out, here are some ideas to consider:

- What day(s) of the week are we most rested?

- Where do we want to go: someplace new or someplace familiar?

- Do we want childcare before or after baby's bedtime?

- How can we ease the pressure to have the perfect night out and enjoy the night that awaits us?

- Who are our favorite people to hang with baby? Which friends would we like to see deepen their relationship with baby?

- How do we want to end our date night?

- Do we each have different desires for our date night? If so, how can we find a win-win?

What Makes This Principle Hard?

The idea of using coregulatory practices to restore your partnership may elicit a giant "Duh! Why *wouldn't* we do that?" But I've noticed two obstacles to making coregulation a daily practice that may be flying under the radar for you. One is the emotional challenge of leaving baby to go out with your partner, the other is cultural. We'll look at how each of these obstacles could be influencing you and your partner, and offer some solutions.

You Don't Want to Leave Baby

There is a palpable emotional pull to be with your baby as often as you can. You love your baby and you love being with your baby. As we've discussed, separations are times of stress for both parents and children. But just because it feels hard doesn't mean leaving is bad for baby or for you guys. Often, the moments of transition are the hardest part. I'm not saying you won't miss baby or baby won't miss you—it's natural to miss those we love most in the world—but you don't have to worry that your bond with your baby will be severed because you and your partner stepped out for some quality time together. In fact, your QT is an opportunity for your little one to develop new bonds. Knowing this buoys me through my own challenges with leaving Jude. I want him to build strong attachment bonds with others in addition to Charlie and me.

What can you do about it? If you find it hard to leave your baby, here are some ways to help you with the separation.

- Find caregivers you'd like to see build relationships with your baby. They may be friends, family, or some of the incredible people who take care of your baby.

- Don't convey your fears to baby. If you're nervous about leaving, your baby will pick up on it. So be sure to introduce caregivers to your baby in a way that shows your trust and support. Notice but don't engage in any subtle ways you might convey fear.

- Remember the importance of putting your own oxygen mask on first. We've talked about the value of caring for yourself and your partnership in order to best care for your child. One form that oxygen mask can take is downtime and activities that recharge you. When I struggle to leave Jude, I use a mantra: *I care for myself so that I can care for Jude.* Feel free to borrow mine or make your own if that helps you.

Coregulation Sounds Like Codependency

"You two are too interconnected and reliant on each other." "Don't be so dependent on your partner." "I need to be able to soothe and excite myself. I shouldn't depend on anyone to do that for me."

In our culture, which values individualism over collaboration, messages warning against dependence abound. We're told to take care of ourselves, first and foremost. So when you hear the guiding principle for this chapter, you might worry that teaming up with your partner at the level of your nervous systems will result in codependency. You might think relying on anyone to care for you in that way is something that parents should do for kids but that adults don't do for each other. You might even fear you'll be less capable of taking care of yourself as a result. Or your partner might have these ideas. Let me be clear: coregulation is not codependency! Nor will it lead to it. Codependency is not based on mutual benefit or equal give and take; rather, one partner relies on the other for their sense of identity. In contrast, coregulation is characterized by mutual care.

What can you do about it? Here are several ways to strengthen your collaboration and ease any worries you or your partner might have about codependency.

- Continually assess whether you and your partner are cared for equally. As long as you both regularly self-assess whether you're being cared for and speak up when you're not, you're engaging in an interdependent relationship, not a codependent one.

- If one of you senses inequity, it's up to both of you to troubleshoot. If one partner says, "This doesn't feeling fair," both partners need to find a solution together. This practice of sharing responsibility for the health of the relationship is itself coregulatory and will produce stronger attachment, safety, and intimacy.

- Don't forget to self-regulate. The first step of the coregulation game in chapter 2 was soothing your own nervous system. Now you and your partner have gone on to become experts on each other, but that doesn't mean you should forget about self-care. There's time for both!

Conclusion

In parenthood—especially early parenthood, when partners' nervous systems are primed for depletion—it's essential for partners to provide themselves with heaps of relationship restoration. To this end, I've shared coregulatory practices for optimum nervous system care. Morning launching and evening landing rituals strengthen your attachment bonds as well as ease your nervous systems during transitions. For more fine-tuning at the nervous system level, I introduced the coregulation station. You experimented with this practice as a way to kick off date nights. You can also use the coregulation station to deepen connection whenever either of you needs some restoration.

Part III of this book, "Thriving in Your Party of Three," begins with the next chapter. In it, we'll cover common struggles, including conflicting responsibilities between family and work, as well as when to begin a career or return to work. And you'll find ways to achieve that ever-elusive balance between family and work life.

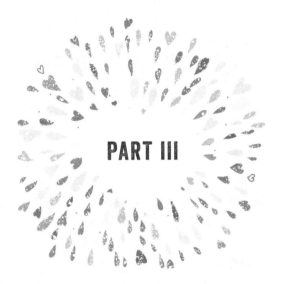

PART III

Thriving in Your Party of Three

CHAPTER 7

Creating Balance

I read Michelle Obama's book *Becoming* when I had about two years of mom status under my belt. For all but four months, I'd been a working mom. Achieving a balance between family and work had been a daily quest for me. Michelle described how, during the sixty minutes she could claim for lunch while working as an executive director, she'd zoom over to a nearby mall, run to various stores and scoop up anything their family needed, then stop at Chipotle for a burrito bowl for herself. Sitting in her car in the strip mall parking lot, eating her burrito bowl and listening to tunes, knowing she'd pulled it off, gave her a sense of delicious accomplishment. Everything and everybody was taken care of.

This scene was so relatable to me—as I imagine it is to most working parents—that I read and reread it and thought about my own eating-Chipotle-in-the-car moments. There was the time I ducked out of a clinical training and scored a private place to pump while I reviewed my notes and ordered new clothes for Jude from my phone—all to the sound of wee-ew-wee-ew-wee-ew. Or all the mornings I amazed myself by taking Jude for a run with me, showering, getting us both dressed, packing our lunches, driving him to school, speaking with his teacher about how he's doing, and still arriving at work with just enough time to do a happy dance before greeting my first client. I would think to myself, *I'm doing this whole working mom life! Everyone is safe and loved!*

Of course, I've had and continue to have many less-than-stellar working mom moments as well. As I reflect on my experience and that of other working parents, I can say with clarity: achieving family and work balance happens in moments. It's not a place of final arrival. You can find and relish balance one day and lose it the next. And you can lose it for reasons totally out of your control. Like sudden demands from your workplace or your child's illness. Or a life-altering global pandemic. If it's not one thing, it's another. In each case, you have to make the effort to find that balance again. In this way, we can consider balance an aspect of secure functioning, which, as you know, exists on a continuum.

To thrive in your party of three, you need solutions that keep your family and work lives balanced on a long-term basis—that serve as a life practice. We start by looking at some dynamics that can throw off that balance; then I give you an exercise to assess how balanced you currently are. A second exercise guides you and your partner to tune up any imbalances, with an eye to creating win-win solutions. Finally, we examine how identifying and committing to family values can amplify the secure-functioning foundation of your family of three.

Guiding Principle 7: You and your partner keep your family and work lives in balance.

The irony that I'm writing a chapter on family and work balance at this particular moment, several weeks into self-quarantining due to the novel coronavirus, is not lost on me. The lines between family life and work have been blurred, and I'm being challenged to find new ways to achieve balance. I'm sitting in the corner of our bedroom, which I've claimed as my new office. Jude just visited to deliver a stuffed snake and request I wear it as I write. The bright pink reptile hanging around my neck reminds me that finding balance is still key in our lives, even in those times when it's damned near impossible to find.

In previous chapters, we've discussed the importance of making decisions mutually and taking care of each other. Creating family and work balance is one specific area where teamwork comes into play. When you're a party of two—and even more as a party of three—that balance can become a complex juggling act.

Besides the dramatic disruption of a pandemic, what kinds of life dynamics can throw your balance off? Let's look at some of the more common ones.

Where you are in your career. If your and your partner's careers are already established when you start your family, taking a step back from work can be a welcome change. If you plan as a team for it, you can take the time you need to readjust your balance as you settle into your party of three. However, maybe you're starting your career and expanding your family during the time frame. Let's say you finished grad school while your baby bomb was ticking, and now you're aching to launch your career. But, you wonder, if childcare is so expensive and you're fresh into your own ability to earn money, will starting work now make sense?

In the absence of secure-functioning teamwork, the demands of a new career alongside the demands of your baby bomb can result in one or the other losing out. To avoid this pressure, some new parents (typically women) decide to postpone their careers. Unless that is a conscious choice made as a team—with a decision-making process in place to identify the eventual right time to start work—it can lead to frustration, resentment, and chronic imbalance.

When to go back to work. Often one or both partners take some time off from work when baby is born. Even if you plan this as a team—including a strategy for achieving balance between your family and work lives—when the time comes, you may find that it's not as easy as you thought. I've already shared the challenge Charlie and I faced when we transitioned from one of us being home with Jude at all times to hiring a sitter so we could both work full time. It's natural to feel anxious about leaving baby and to stress over whether you're completely ready to resume work.

One partner is a stay-at-home parent. One partner functioning as the primary parent and running the household can be a recipe for imbalance. While that work is essential for your party of three, it is *invisible labor*—that is, unpaid and nearly impossible to track or commend. This makes it ripe for misunderstandings and hurt feelings due to lack of appreciation. Even posing the well-intentioned question "What did you do today?" to a stay-at-home parent can backfire emotionally. Work in the home is physically and psychologically demanding, requiring you to continually problem solve ways to care for your child while keeping the house in order. Yet it's not unusual for the house to be completely out of order at the end of the day, which can make it appear as if nothing was accomplished all day.

One partner working too much. When single people work too much, their lack of balance is a choice that affects only them. But if either you or your partner is a workaholic, the other is also affected. And when you become parents, that impact stretches to three and beyond. A heavy work schedule can be inherent in a given job or it can be a habit-driven choice. It can also be a financial necessity. Regardless, it can become a problem if the other partner gets stuck with the brunt of childcare, and you don't have a team process for sorting this out.

One partner parenting too much. Suppose you and your partner both work and have agreed to share parenting responsibilities. Yet you find yourself compelled to pack your daughter's lunch every day because you're convinced your partner isn't up on your child's taste preferences. It's easier to pack the lunch than to discuss this with your partner. You want to let your partner parent more, because you know that's in the best interest of your partnership and your child's well-being. But you can't seem to do it.

The active dominance of one partner who believes they must do it all— either because they are (or believe they are) more capable or because doing it all is critical to their role as a parent—has been called *maternal gatekeeping*. In hetero-partnerships, the woman is usually the one who does this, but because partners of all genders can, I prefer to call it *parental gatekeeping*. Either way, it refers to the micromanaging of childcare, household maintenance, and everything that falls under the parenting umbrella. Doing this pushes your partner out of your team and isolates you from each other.

Too much or too little self-care. Although this chapter is primarily about family and work balance, not all balance issues involve work. How you each take care of yourself also needs to be in balance. Suppose your partner takes up long-distance running post–baby bomb. At first you're thrilled at how happy running makes your partner. His endorphins become the family's endorphins after each run. But then you learn he joined a runners' club. That means he'll be MIA for parent duty several evenings a week, for after-work group runs, and half the day every Saturday, for group runs or races. Your resentment builds as you realize your own self-care will suffer as a result. One partner claiming they don't have any time for self-care isn't any better; martyrdom is bad for the individual and the team. When it comes to balance, too little self-care can be as disruptive as too much.

Balance Check-In

The balance check-in is a tool to help you get a better sense of how balanced your and your partner's family and work scales are. Sit down initially by yourself to answer the questions. For each item, first come up with a number of hours you spend at each activity. Obviously, this should be an estimate. Next, rate your level of enjoyment on a scale of 1 to 10 for that time spent. For example: I spend thirty-five hours a week on my career, and my enjoyment is an 8.

Remember that balance is subjective. What feels good to you may feel off-balance to your partner or your best friend. Try to stay with your own experience here.

How many hours per week do I spend …

- working on my job or career (e.g., commute, time in your workplace, any work you bring home)? Rate your enjoyment level on a scale of 1 to 10.

- working on our home (e.g., cleaning, shopping, household management, laundry, cooking)? Rate your enjoyment level on a scale of 1 to 10.

- being with my partner, just the two of us (e.g., at home or out on the town)? Rate your enjoyment level on a scale of 1 to 10.

- being with our child (e.g., childcare, transportation, playdates, meals, activities, and lessons)? Rate your enjoyment level on a scale of 1 to 10.

- on self-care? Rate your enjoyment level on a scale of 1 to 10.

After you've collected your data, I suggest writing about it in your journal to get a deeper understanding about what this means for you as an individual and what it means for your partnership. Note that this isn't a one-time deal; I recommend doing periodic balance check-ins, especially as circumstances change in your life.

Your partner can also do the exercise on their own. In the next exercise, which I call a "balance tune-up," you two will have an opportunity to share your check-in results and negotiate a win-win for any areas that are out of balance.

Balancing as a Team

Patrick scoops some toys off the sofa and motions to Danny to sit next to him. "Etta's asleep, so how about we go over our balance check-ins?"

"I know she's asleep. I just put her down," Danny says coolly as he drops onto the sofa and reaches for his tablet. "I can tell you right off—my scores aren't high."

Patrick looks over Danny's results and compares them with the scores on his own tablet. While all of his own enjoyment scores are high, Danny's are another story. "Look at job and career," he says. "We have a big imbalance there. I rated my enjoyment a 10, and you gave yours a 1."

"And look at the imbalance of hours for working on our home," Danny says.

"Well, that's no surprise since you're home full time," Patrick says. "What I don't get is why your enjoyment of it is only a 2. And your enjoyment of being with Etta is only a 5, and your self-care is at a 1. Dude! What on earth is going on here?"

"Obviously I enjoy being with Etta. I *love* being with her," Danny says. "But when I added up my hours, it really hit home—with all the work I do around here, I'll be a senior citizen before I go back to school. That's the reason for my low scores."

Patrick is genuinely surprised. "I didn't realize you still wanted to go back to school."

"Of course I do. Did you think my goal of getting into health care evaporated when we adopted Etta? She's three years old, and I've been putting that dream on hold—and carrying a heavier load than you—for far too long!"

"A heavier load than *me?*" Patrick stares down at the seventy hours he proudly recorded for his real estate job. He feels lightheaded from the mix of alarm and anger flooding through him. "You can't be serious? For three years I've been sacrificing my time with you and Etta so we can live in this lovely home—this home you hate to work on!"

"I couldn't be more serious," Danny says. "It hurt to write down those low scores. You don't need to spend seventy hours at work, you could slow down and spend more time with Etta. Maybe it wasn't such a good idea to do this balance check-in."

Patrick is still in shock. He sits there, silently shaking his head, thinking, *I don't see how we get past this without one of us being a big loser.*

♥♥♥

Neither partner in this scenario can see this discussion as the beginning of a satisfying redistribution of labor. They aren't working as a team yet. They're taking their scores at face value and leaving it at that. Completing the balance check-in provides data on how you spend your time and how you feel about it.

But that's not enough. Your next step is to get with your partner, listen to each other, figure out why some of your scores are low, and troubleshoot a solution together.

One of you may be out of balance in your life, both of you might be out of balance in your lives, and you might be out of balance with each other. All three of these—or a combination thereof—are possible. If one of you is out of balance, the other can provide support. For example, if the only insight gained from this exercise was that Patrick wanted to spend less time at work, they could have focused on brainstorming solutions to that. It's more tricky when the imbalance is at the relationship level. Then you need to find a win-win solution. Remember, win-wins are solutions both partners feel positive about; neither partner walks away from a win-win feeling resentment or harboring hurt feelings.

Win-wins are a hallmark of secure-functioning relationships. You two recognize that the more balanced each of you feels, the better off your partnership is. So it's not totally selfless—it's actually in your self-interest to care about your partner's balance or lack thereof. This is the bedrock of secure functioning: you both want what's good for both of you. It's the ultimate in teamwork. And it makes your partnership a place where both of you want to be, a place that feels good to both of your nervous systems and brings glowing yellow security into your lives.

Balance Tune-Up

Sit down with your partner to compare your balance check-in results and discuss how you each feel about your respective time and enjoyment scores.

1. Take turns sharing your own ratings. This is where listening is key. Take your partner at their word if they don't feel good about the equity in your partnership. Give each other the benefit of the doubt. The tips for constructive communication I've already shared with you apply here too: be open and honest, be direct, be respectful and kind, practice sherlocking, self-assess, and coregulate.

2. Discuss your ratings. Here are some questions to ask each other:

    •   In general, do we as a couple have a good balance between family and work?

- Is one of us spending more time than we wish in any area? Less time?

- How do our respective hours and ratings match up for each question?

- Are any of our ratings 5 or lower? What might that indicate?

3. Negotiate a win-win. Pick one or two ways in which you feel out of balance, either individually or as a couple. Find some solutions to better balance work and family. They must be win-wins.

Revisiting Patrick and Danny

Let's see how Patrick and Danny look when they follow their check-in with a balance tune-up.

"This is really gonna take some sorting out, love," Danny says as he sets the baby monitor down and passes his tablet to Patrick. "I have lousy scores in nearly every area."

Patrick looks Danny in the eyes and sees his husband is pretty down. "Don't worry. We'll figure this out." After the two of them have reviewed their scores, he says, "What do you know about your low scores, Danny?"

This question helps Danny focus, and he starts to feel a bit better. "When I was journaling, I discovered how bummed I am about not following my life goals. I really want to be a nurse practitioner."

"Wow! I'm so happy to hear you still want to do that. You'd make a great nurse, Danny!" Patrick says.

"Thanks," Danny says, blushing. "My dream has always been to help others. I'm glad I spent these years with Etta, but I'm ready to shift. And I'm going to need your help."

"Okay," Patrick says, with a hard swallow.

Danny immediately spots Patrick's tell. "I see you tightening. What's going on?"

"I can't get away with anything in front of you!" Patrick smiles, overriding his slight annoyance at Danny's good sherlocking skills.

Danny smiles back. "I'm here to know you and love you, babe."

This touches Patrick, and he starts to relax. "I need your help too. Now that we're digging into this, those seventy hours I clock at work are starting to feel out of whack with the twelve I spend with Etta. I don't know how you're going to react to this, but … I want to work less and spend more time with her."

"Why would that bother me? I love that idea!" Danny exclaims.

Patrick likes this straight-up enthusiasm but wants to be up front about their challenges. "It means less money for our family. And school will be expensive."

"Oh, Patrick!" Danny reaches for his husband's hand so it's clear what he's about to say isn't a criticism but is in the spirit of a team win-win. "You always think you have to do everything for our family. I'll look into student loans and grants, no worries! Plus, if you pull back at work, you can watch Etta more, which will cut down on childcare. This is exactly the tune-up we need."

Patrick relaxes deeply, his head resting on Danny's shoulder. "Good, cause I'm a bit freaked. You know how I am with change."

Danny laughs. "I do. But this will be better for all three of us. Etta will be happy to be with you more, and I think it's good for her to see me work outside the home too."

❤❤❤

As you can see, these partners are well on their way to finding win-wins for their family of three. They care as much about each other's scores as they do about their own. They are able to coregulate and use their status as experts on each other to diffuse tensions, allowing them to find their way into yellow security and openness together.

Note that key to their success is their willingness to probe what is underneath their low scores (Patrick wanting to spend more time with Etta, Danny wanting to go back to school). It can take some effort, both alone and together, to get to the reason for low scores and find a win-win, so don't give up on the process if it doesn't work the first time around. Plan for multiple discussions as you make these joint decisions. Your goal is to create an infrastructure for balance, and that's a big endeavor.

Secure-Functioning Family Values

You and your partner may be able to readily improve the balance of your family and work lives by negotiating win-wins. But what if you can't? If achieving balance is a challenge—or if you simply want to go deeper in your efforts to build a balanced foundation for your party of three—examining the values you hold as a family can help.

Many of our values come from our first family or from the culture we grew up in. Often we imbibe these values unconsciously. As adults, we may not realize what some of our values are; all we know is that we have strong feelings about how those values play out day to day. This is compounded in a relationship if we also don't know all of our partner's values.

Despite both working full time, a couple I'll call Mia and Remy couldn't find a way to cut costs so they could afford to send their son to a different preschool, something they both wanted. They had been at loggerheads over this for a while when Mia spotted a large expense on their bank statement. "What's *this?*"

"That's my black credit card!" Remy was immediately defensive.

"Do you realize how much its $5,000 annual fee would help with preschool?"

Remy couldn't deny that. But he didn't see a possible win-win. "I'll look like a total nobody if I can't slap down my black card when I'm with clients!" he wailed.

Mia thought she knew her partner, but this stunned her. "Babe, you're not a nobody! You're the best dad, the best partner, the best sales rep!"

♥♥♥

This exchange led to a revelation for the couple. As they explored the values underlying their respective positions, it became clear that what Remy considered a necessary status symbol for his work, Mia saw as an unnecessary expense for their family. Both were carrying on values they learned growing up. In this case, Remy came to agree that saving money was an important value for their new family, especially given the economic uncertainties in the wider world. He and Mia were able to talk out what they want to hold as family values going forward.

When you hear me stress the term *family values,* you may find yourself wincing. It may evoke uncomfortable thoughts about so-called traditional family values, whereby the nuclear family is the only valued structure, and within that structure, women stay home, and men bring home the bacon. And it's true: the term has been politicized and used to exclude some people and ways of living. I'd like us to reclaim it. Rather than using it to value one family structure over another, we can use it to refer to the set of values that bring your family of three into alignment—regardless of the structure of your family.

In chapter 5, we talked about valuing your needs individually and as partners. Here, we go deeper to clarify not just the needs you value but the core values that hold your family together and support your secure functioning. Some of these values may overlap with what you consider needs, while others may be more broadly defined as beliefs, principles, or standards. Common values for families include many things:

- hard work and financial success
- life-long learning
- good physical and mental health
- time together as a family or with your child
- personal alone time and alone time as a couple
- a network of friends
- extended family
- travel
- nature
- religion or spirituality
- loyalty
- honesty
- integrity
- open-mindedness
- balance itself can be a value!

Note that some common values may presuppose the privilege that allows you to even consider them. For example, the ability to travel long distances may be limited by your child's age or a pandemic; where your child attends school may be driven by financial considerations. If you feel something you value is out of reach for you right now, dig deeper and ask what specifically you value about it. In the case of travel, you might value diverse cultural experiences. In the case of school choice, you might value lifelong learning. Use those deeper values to refine your list.

DISCOVER AND CLAIM YOUR VALUES

You can do this exercise by yourself or together with your partner.

1. Find a quiet time to ask yourself these questions:

    *   What is important to me in raising a child? In being a partner? In being a person in the world?

    *   Where did these values come from?

    *   Do I want to carry these values forward, or do I want to reconsider any of them?

2. From the values you identified in step 1, pick five you consider core family values. For each, answer the following questions:

    *   Do my partner and I share this family value?

    *   Did we consciously choose this family value?

    *   Does this value support our secure functioning as a family?

    *   Are we proud of this as our family value?

    *   Do we consistently act on this value in our family?

If you and your partner do this exercise together, you may want to revisit your couple agreement from chapter 3 and make sure it reflects your family values in all the ways you'd like.

What Makes This Principle Hard?

Creating balance can sometimes feel like you're trying to hit a moving target. Chances are you'll feel imbalanced in some way at some point, and that experience will force you and your partner on a journey to find balance. As you attempt to clarify your family values as part of that journey, one obstacle you may encounter is the cultural narrative around traditional family values. This is especially true if yours is a nontraditional family. Another challenge that can make finding balance hard is the persistent inequality between women and men in the workplace. Let's examine these issues and some solutions.

Family Values Are Outdated

"First comes marriage, then comes baby in a baby carriage." "The mommy wars: you're either a good mom who stay homes or a good feminist who works outside the home." "Children need to be raised by a mom and a dad; two moms or two dads is harmful."

Even hearing that the family values I'm talking about are in no way limited to traditional values, you may still feel put off. For so long, you've heard the messaging of mainstream culture that wants you to think a nontraditional family's values are somehow different from or inferior to other families' values. I'm here to say, not so! *All* families can claim their values and allow those values to guide them in blazing their own paths.

"Family values" is not the first co-opted term that needs to be reclaimed in our culture, and I'm sure it won't be the last. For example, "wholesome" was traditionally used to promote chastity, and women who waited until marriage to have sex were called "wholesome." It became a weapon against women, using their sexuality to keep them in their place. More recently, an advertising campaign helped flip this script by using "wholesome" to refer to minority, blended, and LGBTQ families. As a result, "wholesome" has a newly inclusive meaning in our culture.

What can you do about it? The best way to counter the old stereotypes around family values is to come up with your own values and proudly call them family values. You and your partner can help reclaim the term simply by using it and being inclusive. Talk to your friends and family about your family values and ask them about theirs. Hopefully, with all our efforts, it will make its way into the cultural zeitgeist in a new and radical way.

The Motherhood Penalty

Let's be blunt: misogyny and sexism are alive and well in the workplace. Some people might like to focus on the progress that's been made, but the cold hard fact is that gender inequalities persist. Women still earn less than men. Census Bureau stats tell us white women earn 82 cents on the dollar compared with men. For women of color, it is even less—as low as 54 cents for Latinas.

These disparities are fed by misogyny and discrimination—latent or overt or both.

How does this relate to your baby bomb? It turns out, the baby bomb plays a significant role in the form of what has been called the *motherhood penalty.* Studies by the U.S. Census Bureau show that becoming parents increases gender pay inequities. In the year after their baby bomb, the earnings gap between partners in hetero relationships doubles. Working mothers earn only 71 cents for every dollar paid to working fathers. In addition, because many moms take on the lion's share of home and child responsibilities, lack of affordable childcare hinders moms more than dads.

What starts out as an imbalance in the workplace can translate into a felt imbalance at home. One partner earning less or having to work harder for the same pay can put a strain on the relationship. It also highlights the critical need for childcare to better balance your family and work lives. Unfortunately, our society doesn't provide parents with childcare, and many parents struggle to afford it.

What can you do about it? If you feel passionate about correcting gender inequities in the workplace, consider upping your activism game and supporting those who have plans to change government policies about parental leave and about quality, affordable childcare. If you're in a hetero couple, be alert to the subtle and not-so-subtle ways the inequalities that exist in the world at large creep into your relationship. Both of you are responsible for continual assessment at home so you give equal value to each other's work—even if society does not—and make sure the patriarchy doesn't undermine your partnership. In the words of Ruth Bader Ginsburg, "Women will only have true equality when men share with them the responsibility of bringing up the next generation."

At the same time, we need to acknowledge that childcare and other support systems will not always be available. Your income may not allow you to hire a sitter when you want some child-free time for balance. Or the village you create might not be available for reasons beyond anyone's control. When no one can step in to lend a hand, don't give up on balance. Instead, learn to create it in innovative ways.

What might that look like? For me, as I mentioned, the other day it looked like a stuffed toy, a pink snake, hanging around my neck. But it wasn't just the snake. When the pandemic hit, Charlie and I put our heads together to figure out how we could rise to this new challenge and balance our lives. He had a project with a pressing deadline, so we agreed I would use my working hours to see clients and would postpone writing time so I could watch Jude while Charlie finished that project. We both had to make sacrifices and couldn't achieve the level of balance we normally like; nevertheless, it was a win-win in the situation. We also made sure I wasn't paying the motherhood penalty in our marriage.

When you and your partner have limited childcare options, negotiate a win-win. Discuss what each of you is willing to sacrifice and for how long. As long as you do this as a team, it will be a win-win. Your teamwork becomes the cushion that softens the sacrifice.

Conclusion

The ability to create balance is foundational to the secure functioning of your family of three. Especially if you're experiencing conflicting responsibilities between family and work, wondering when to begin your career or return to work, or struggling to maintain a precarious sense of balance, you want to check in with yourself and with your partner to assess how balanced your lives are. You also want to get with your partner on a regular basis to tune up any imbalances and negotiate win-win solutions. You can go deeper by identifying and committing to family values that amplify your secure-functioning foundation.

One area of your relationship that can easily get out of balance as you adjust to your baby bomb is sex. In the next chapter, we look at the multitude of changes that can occur in sexual activity and desire when baby arrives. You will learn ways to keep romance alive in the face of these challenges.

CHAPTER 8

Finding a New Spring of Sexuality

A couple of months after Jude was born, Charlie approached me in our bedroom one afternoon, after I'd put Jude down for a nap, and initiated sex for the first time since we had become parents.

I was stunned. There we were, in our bedroom, a place we'd been intimate countless times before, but the idea of having sex felt completely foreign to me. I thought, *Oh yeah, people do that; people have sex. I used to have sex! And I used to like having sex!* It hadn't occurred to me till that very moment to miss sex, let alone feel sexual. It was as if a desire valve had been shut off in me from the moment I became a mom, and I hadn't even noticed. I looked back at Charlie, my nonexistent poker face full of surprise. Blushing slightly, with a tinge of self-consciousness, I said, "I don't know if I'm up for that ...."

I paused to check in with myself. Along with shock and surprise—and the realization I couldn't yet imagine using my body for my own pleasure again—I also felt gratitude for Charlie's willingness to reach out. Still, it was clear to me that just the suggestion of sex was enough for today. I said, "Not right now, but thank you for suggesting it."

Reestablishing a healthy sex life post–baby bomb can be a journey. That day, Charlie and I began ours. It was and continues to be the full rainbow of experiences—fits and starts, awkwardness, tears of joy, emotional connectedness, and grief. Finding time and space for desire to bloom took care, patience, and mutual understanding. I wouldn't have had it any other way, because this journey has added a new depth of intimacy and trust to our partnership.

Sexuality can be such an essential part of life, a sacred way to communicate with and show love for your partner. For most couples, rocking and rolling as a team means having an active sex life you both enjoy. And you both get to define what *active* means for you. Every couple is different in terms of frequency of sex, actual time spent being intimate, what constitutes intimacy, and so on. There is no "right" sex life. There is only the one you both enjoy.

Perhaps you've noticed that life post–baby bomb without sex can turn into a very long winter. This chapter's guiding principle helps you find your way back to springtime as you reclaim romance and intimate connection. Because birthing mothers undergo such dramatic physical and psychological transformations, I emphasize their experience. However, all parents can find support here—parents adopting children, same-sex parents using a surrogate, non-birthing moms in same-sex relationships, as well as dads in hetero relationships.

We begin with a discussion of the physical issues that can interfere with sex, including hormonal changes, healing from the birth, and fatigue. Then we look at sexual connection from a psychological lens, examining how your view of your body affects sexual intimacy, as well as what happens in your and your partner's minds when romance fades in early parenthood.

Guiding Principle 8: You and your partner redefine romance to keep your couple connection alive.

Often, though not always, the pleasure of sex is what brings babies into our lives. Yet having and enjoying sex post–baby bomb is something most couples need to work at—or at the very least, be thoughtful about—to successfully bring it back into their partnerships. Why is this? Birthing moms go through massive physical and psychological changes during pregnancy and early postpartum life. Also, non-birthing partners experience the aftermath of lack of sleep, their own changes in identity, fears (or the reality) of being rejected repeatedly when initiating intimacy, and struggles to find the time and energy for sex. All this takes a toll. In a study of first-time Irish moms by Deirdre O'Malley and colleagues, nearly half reported a lack of interest in sexual activity as much as six months after giving birth, and the percentage was not much lower at one year.

It's easy to see how sex can get put on the back burner when so much else is going on during early parenthood. But keeping it on the back burner can become problematic for your well-being and that of your coupledom. One solution is to re-envision how you see romance. Pre–baby bomb, romance might have looked like spontaneously grabbing a bottle of good wine, silencing your devices, and having some fun time between the sheets. That's no longer your daily reality. You need a new definition of romance that allows you two to connect intimately, emotionally, sensually, and supportively with each other as you are in the present moment. What does that look like? One new mom I know captured it when she said to her partner, "The most romantic thing you could do for me right now is … the laundry." You laugh, but she was being honest. And to his credit, her partner understood that they needed to connect in new ways.

This guiding principle asks you to redefine romance to include whatever brings you connection. Let's look first at the physical impact of a baby bomb for birthing mothers and then at its psychological impact. In each section, we'll focus on what you can do to regenerate Eros.

Physical Impact

Starting with pregnancy, having a baby and caring for a young child have a huge impact on birthing mamas' bodies. Even if you don't anticipate it, some of these experiences dramatically change you. Although there are many types of physical impact, let's look at three that can cause radical change: hormones, the birth event, and fatigue.

The Hormone Storm

During my pregnancy and early postpartum life, my hormones felt like giant swells building inside me, amplifying whatever feeling I was having. When I was happy, I was ecstatic. When I was sad, I was gutted. When I was frustrated, I felt explosive.

In my first trimester, I drove to a wolf sanctuary to speak with the director about a workshop I was scheduled to teach later that year. The bright Southern California sun and blue sky filled me with hope and optimism. After meeting the director, I spent time with the wolves. I was especially drawn to Maya, the matriarch of the pack. When she came up and gently nuzzled my belly, I intuited that she knew I had a hitchhiker in there. I imagined she was blessing Jude with her supreme wolf wisdom. I cried with happiness the whole way home, my heart pounding with delight. I'm prone to big feelings, but my happiness that day felt drenched in hormones.

During pregnancy, you experience an increase in estrogen and progesterone. After birth, those hormones are replaced with an oxytocin surge. The milk-making hormone prolactin, which makes breastfeeding possible, also surges. When you wean your baby, prolactin fades, giving your body yet another hormonal shift.

All birthing mothers may have the same basic hormone shifts, but each woman's experience is different. After Charlie initiated sex on that first afternoon, I reflected on why my desire was on mute and traced it back to hormones. Some women's desire increases with their pregnancy hormone surge, while others' desire decreases. Post–baby bomb, although hormones take about a month to return to pre-pregnancy levels, women take varying amounts of time to rekindle their interest in sex. Ultimately, it doesn't matter how your hormones affect you per se; what's important is how aware are you of their impact, how aware your partner is, and how you help each other redefine romance so you can connect.

Here are some healing tips for birthing moms:

- Recognize your own swell of hormones. Are you not feeling like yourself? Feeling "off" or "odd" is a clue that something may be up with your hormones.

- Find your own way to ride the waves. Ask yourself, "What kind of support do I need right now?" It may be extra TLC from your partner or a friend or just taking time for yourself.

- Let the voice of your hormones guide how you experience romance. Some days you may need cuddles, care, and a shoulder to cry on; other days, a pillow fight can release tension.

- Communicate in an ongoing way about your experience so your partner is aware and can become a source of support. Let your partner be the ally you need.

Here are some healing tips for non-birthing partners:

- Recognize that your partner's body is undergoing a massive change inside. Just because you can't see some changes doesn't make them less significant.

- Ask often how your partner is doing. This builds an ease between the two of you so you can talk about all the internal changes as they occur.

- Listen to your partner. If your partner is struggling and upset about something you don't consider a big deal, don't lead with your judgment.

- Discover and create new ways to experience romantic connection.

The Birth Event

Belly and vaginal births are full-on physical events that can be traumatic for the birthing mom's body. Injuries from childbirth are incredibly common, including injuries to the pelvic floor (which can occur during both belly and vaginal births), vaginal tearing or episiotomies, and cesarean section discomfort and tightness. These injuries can have major ripple effects in your sex life for quite some time.

I believe one thing that makes it hard for birthing mamas to think about sex again is that most of us don't have a space in which the birth event can be metabolized and healed in a loving way. Think of that infamous six-week postpartum checkup. Mine only covered a sliver of recovery: a postpartum depression assessment, an exam that revealed I was physically ready for sex and exercise, and a discussion about what birth control I planned to use while nursing Jude. Those three topics were important, but they missed the full impact birthing had on me. So much of the physical impact of childbirth is unspoken and unattended to, which can have a domino effect on sexual desire.

Here are some healing tips for birthing moms:

- Talk about how your body is doing. I suggest talking with your doctor as well as your partner, friends, and family. Consider joining a moms' group.

- Tell your birth story as many times as you need to. This will help you arrive at a cohesive narrative that is critical to emotional healing.

- Be gentle with your body as it heals. Go easy on physical labor. Take long baths and spend time connecting with your body. You can deepen this practice by noticing your inhales and exhales while you're submerged in water.

- If you can afford it, get bodywork (physical therapy, massage, acupuncture) from providers who specialize in postpartum healing.

Here are some healing tips for non-birthing partners:

- Recognize that your partner is healing from a physically dramatic event. Don't underestimate the time and space that may be needed for full healing.

- Ask often how your partner is doing. Listen attentively.

- Support your partner taking the time to physically heal. Encourage your partner to engage in self-care and, if needed, to seek out professional support.

- Step up for childcare and household chores (and yes, do the laundry).

Fatigue

The most fatigued I've ever felt was when Jude was six months old. I had run out of new-parent adrenaline and excitement to push me through the days. All I had left was rocket-fuel strong coffee and my hope this would pass so I could someday get more sleep again. Jude was in the middle of a gnarly four-month sleep regression, which had started around the time I went back to work, and I was up with him every ninety minutes at night. I was tired to the bone. And the fatigue was cumulative. I was putting-socks-away-in-the-refrigerator tired. I was forgetting-which-breast-I'd-fed-Jude-with-and-developing-a-clot tired. I was wearing-my-nursing-bra-and-swimsuit-bottom-to-Jude's-swim-class tired. Even my hair was tired.

Early parenthood is physically exhausting. Birthing mamas are physically recovering from childbirth at the same time that they're already sleep deprived. Non-birthing partners are also physically tired. A study of German parents by David Richter and colleagues reported it took parents six years to fully recover from sleep deprivation and feel like they were getting satisfactory sleep again. Six years! Not feeling rested most definitely diminishes your sexual desire and ability to enjoy sex.

Here are some healing tips for birthing moms:

- Claim rest when you can. Parents are advised to "sleep when baby sleeps," but you can't always do that. If you can't sleep when baby sleeps, rest instead. Just lying down and closing your eyes is restorative.

- Remind yourself that this is a phase, and sleep is on the horizon.

- Reframe romance. For example, think of your partner giving you a chance to get quality rest as them giving you a bouquet of roses.

- Talk to your partner about taking turns on night duty for baby. Even if you want to wake and pump for milk supply reasons, try to take a night off.

Here are some healing tips for non-birthing partners:

- Claim rest when you can. Fill up your cup when the water (i.e., downtime from parenting and work) is flowing.

- Offer to help with night duty. When it's your night, don't wake your partner for help unless you absolutely need to.

- Look for new ways to create romance with your partner.

Psychological Impact

A friend once described the psychological changes of becoming a parent as so massive that it was like becoming a new gender. All this upheaval can cause disarray in your erotic life. In this section, we consider two major points of impact: body image (i.e., how you view and feel about the shape of your body) and the sustained loss of intimate romantic connection that can be hard to come back from.

Body Change Blues

Iris scans her closet, looking for clothes she could feel sexy in. As she makes her way through the hangers, her heart sinks. "I remember when I could rock this," she says, pulling out a fitted maxi summer dress. "Now my breasts will pour out the top. That is, if I can even get it zipped." She lets out a big sigh.

Mark comes into the bedroom just in time to hear Iris mention her breasts pouring out. "Hey, you're exactly where I want you!" he says, making his way over to her.

Iris doesn't even look toward him. She's still staring at the clothes in her closet. "I think I'll start bagging some of these for charity. No sense having them take up space when I can't wear them."

"Sure," Mark says as he puts an arm around her waist and squeezes.

Iris turns quickly toward him. "What're you doing?" she asks, visibly irritated.

"God forbid I try to put my arm around my wife!"

"I'm having a moment, Mark. Can't you see I'm not in the mood?"

Mark jumps back, stung. "You're never in the mood! Katrina will be in kindergarten before I see you naked again."

Iris looks at him with disgust. "You put the moves on me when I'm damn near crying about not fitting into my clothes, and you expect me to rejoice at this opportunity for sex? Where is Katrina anyway?"

"In her crib. Don't change the subject. We need to talk about why we're not having sex. Touch is my love language. I need it."

Iris prickles at the pressure for sex she feels from Mark. "I'll have sex with you when I'm ready. In the meantime, please don't touch me like that."

"Fine. I'll never touch you again!" Mark storms out of the bedroom and heads back to Katrina's room. He smiles when he sees her playing in her crib, but his heart is heavy. *Maybe she's not into me anymore,* he thinks. *Maybe she just doesn't find me attractive now that I'm a dad.*

Meanwhile, Iris is tossing half her wardrobe onto the bed. *I can't imagine what it'll take to feel sexy again,* she thinks. *My body is so different now. I wish Mark understood that. I feel so lonely.*

♥♥♥

Both Iris and Mark feel like they're the only new parents in the world not connecting sexually. Iris feels like she's the only new mom with a body she doesn't like or understand anymore. But these two aren't alone. Case in point, the research I mentioned earlier on first-time Irish moms found that being dissatisfied with their body image was a significant factor behind lack of interest in sex a full year postpartum. In another study, Elise Riquin and her colleagues found that moms who were unhappy about their physical appearance were four times more likely than other moms to have postnatal depression.

If you're struggling to feel comfortable in your body, understand that there's nothing wrong with you. What you're feeling is normal, and there are ways you can shift your body image. One place to turn is toward what we know from attachment theory. As we saw in chapter 1, people on the yellow secure range of the attachment continuum tend to be comfortable with themselves, including with their body image. Blue and red peeps tend to be less comfortable, and the dramatic physical changes of pregnancy can accentuate their discomfort. Moreover, whatever color you are, remember that big events themselves can move you on the continuum. Even if you were yellow before, the birth of your child can push you into red or blue and turn up feelings of shame and dislike for your body shape.

The first step in improving your body image is to understand that your comfort level with your body is a product of your ability for secure functioning. It has nothing to do with the actual shape or size of your body, and making decisions that affect its size or shape should be based on health, not image. It's not about having the "perfect" body; the "perfect" body doesn't exist, and trying to create one will not give you comfort in your own skin. There's no such thing as a yellow secure body. What is yellow is the security that comes from your own acceptance of your body as it is. You move toward yellow on the continuum by practicing acceptance of your body.

The second step is to use your secure-functioning team to solidify your acceptance of your body image. The non-birthing partner can support the birthing partner's move toward greater acceptance. Let's see how Iris and Mark do this.

This time, as Iris scans her closet for clothes she could feel sexy in, she pulls out her fitted maxi summer dress. "I remember when I could rock this, and my breasts wouldn't pour out," she says to herself.

Mark comes into the bedroom and catches Iris talking to herself. "Hey babe, you're rocking it in those overalls right now!" he says, making his way over to her.

Iris looks at him and laughs. "I'm glad you think so."

"That's cause you are sexy and will always be. To me anyway!" Mark says. Then he notices Iris isn't laughing anymore. Her eyes look a little watery as she stares at the dress. He puts his hand gently on her waist and say, "How're you feeling, babe?"

She steps away from him and plunks down on the bed. "Honestly? I'm frustrated with my body. I'm frustrated that it's taking so long to get back to normal. If normal even exists anymore. Maybe I should give these old clothes to charity."

"You could do that." Mark sits on the bed a couple feet from Iris, sensing she needs a little physical distance as she processes her feelings about her body.

Iris senses Mark's support. If he had insisted she keep the clothes, that would have felt like pressure to get her body to do things it can't right now. "I might actually do that," she says. "Some of them anyway."

"Make a little more space for your sexy new-mom clothes," Mark says, his eyes smiling encouragement as he twangs the strap on her overalls.

"Thanks, love. I need your help with this. I won't be mad if you tell me every day how super sexy I am," Iris says, smiling back. She picks up the summer dress and folds it neatly. "I think I'll donate this in Katrina's honor. My body wouldn't be the size it is now if it weren't for our darling daughter."

RECONNECTING WITH YOUR EROTIC SELF

The first three steps of this exercise are specifically for birthing moms to do alone, but both partners can complete all four steps. Body image doesn't only affect one gender; often both partners have painful body image issues to heal. Because the journey toward body acceptance is ongoing, I suggest making this exercise a regular practice.

1. Spend some time gazing at your naked body in a mirror. Look yourself over from head to toe. You may notice areas of your body you're hesitant to look at or want to avoid completely. Try to look at these areas. Visually take in your entire body.

2. Grab your journal and write down all the thoughts, images, and random words that came up while gazing at your body. Do this in a free-association style. Then journal about the following questions:

    •   How do I see my body?

    •   How do I think about my body?

    •   How do I feel about my body?

- How do I act with my partner as a result?

3. Offer gratitude. Your body has been through a lot. Finish your journaling session by making a list of the things you're grateful to your body for.

4. Grab your partner for a game of What I Love About Your Body. Sit face to face and take turns picking a body part of the other and saying what you love about it. This might sound like "I love how your shoulders ..." or "What I love about your breasts is ..." or "I love your eyes because ..." or "I love the freckle on the underside ..." See if you can redefine romance, body part by body part.

Romance Blues

If it's been a long time since you and your partner enjoyed sex or eroticism, you may have fallen into a romance rut. Even if you think you're ready to end the long winter, you can't just snap your fingers and say, "It's spring now—let's start having sex again." Often partners who haven't been intimate with each other for a long while build psychological walls that make it harder to rekindle romance. We saw this with Mark and Iris. When he threatened, "I'll never touch you again," he was letting Iris know he had lost confidence in their ability to connect intimately. Iris confirmed similar feelings when she thought, *I feel so lonely.* We discussed how this couple could begin healing Iris's body image blues, but in reality, they would likely also need to address their overarching romance blues.

Like body image blues, romance blues grow out of the inability to be a secure-functioning team during the tumultuous transition into parenthood. Your minds can weave convincing stories that keep you and your partner in a snowy winter. Like Mark, your story can be something along the lines of *She doesn't think my being a dad is sexy. If I touch her again, she'll just reject me. So I won't even try.* Or it can be like Iris: *I'm not desirable anymore. This is what being a mom is like. So I'm just going to forget sex, because I've lost that part of me anyway.* If your story and your partner's story reinforce each other, then breaking the narrative can be even more challenging.

Many factors can feed your narrative. For example, it can be intimating to initiate sex if you've been rejected several times. Or you can feel vulnerable sharing your body when it almost doesn't feel like your body anymore, due to all its changes. Or being out of practice can make you and your partner feel shy.

The best way out of the romance blues is different for different couples. I'm going to offer three exercises, each with a different focus. Feel free to try any or all of them, depending on what resonates.

Sex Every Day

Sometimes, even if there's a lot going on under the surface, I find it can work for couples to not overthink it and just welcome in spring. You can take the pressure off reigniting romantic intimacy by making an agreement to have sex every day for a period of time. If you and your partner are both up for it, agreeing to be naked between the sheets every day can take away uncertainty and performance anxiety.

1. Discuss the terms of your agreement. How long are you committing to this experiment? It could be sex every day for one week, two weeks, ten days, a month, or whatever you guys feel is doable.

2. Also discuss what "counts" as sex: do you expect to have intercourse every day or is cuddling naked okay on some days?

3. Discuss how you'll handle it if one of you needs to take the day off for whatever reason. Consider if you want to add a day to the experiment or simply skip a day.

4. Agree that you both will be equal initiators of sex. No one person is responsible to initiate each day; it's on both of you to keep your agreement.

Scheduling Sex

One challenge as you try to reignite your romance is that the logistics are different now that baby's here. Remember when you could give each other a look and have sex in the kitchen? Or on the couch? Or in the car? That freedom is in your rearview mirror. So instead of flashing forward twenty years to when you'll have your home to yourselves again, consider this exercise: scheduling sex.

Before you reject this as too mechanical or unspontaneous, give it a try. Many couples find that scheduling sex is an aphrodisiac in itself. One couple I know start texting each other while at work. One will suggest a time for sex, and they have fun building their excitement throughout the day until the main event. They say that in some ways, sex is better than it was pre–baby bomb, because now the whole day of anticipation brings big rewards.

COLLABORATIVE STORIES

What if you and your partner aren't quite ready for sex every day or scheduling sex? The stories you've been telling yourselves about why you aren't having sex or why your partner doesn't find you sexy might have taken root a bit too firmly to just set them aside without another thought. If this is the case, I recommend an exercise based on a technique Stan uses to help couples move toward secure functioning.

You and your partner can do this as a game. The idea is that you start by listening to each other's stories and then build a collaborative story.

1. Find some quiet time to sit down together. First take turns telling each other your current story about sex—including any fears you have about rejection, performance anxiety, lack of sexiness, and so on. To do this successfully, you have to (a) be completely open and honest in telling your story, and (b) listen nonjudgmentally to your partner's story.

2. Listen without judgment. It might be tempting to correct your partner at this point ("But you *are* sexy!" "I never meant to reject you!"). Hold off on that for now. Just listen to each other's current stories and make a note of how similar or different they are.

3. Now tell each other a second story: describe what you want for your sexual relationship. It can be as juicy as you wish.

4. Compare you second stories. How collaborative are they? Can you take these stories into the bedroom?

What Makes This Principle Hard?

Redefining romance to fan your couple connection post–baby bomb takes thoughtful work. Even though this work is fun, you can run into your fair share of obstacles. One potential obstacle is the diet culture and all its harmful messaging. Another is the phenomenon of *over touch*. Let's look at these issues a bit more closely and find some solutions.

Diet Culture Shames You

"What are you going to do about that mom pooch?" "Ten ways to get the pre-baby sexy you back!" "Real ways to lose the weight while breastfeeding." "Shred the weight and be a happy mom!"

Diet culture is an insidious belief system that emphasizes the value of thinness over health and emotional well-being. The dieting industry targets women from a young age with the message that being thin is the key to beauty, happiness, and sexuality. By the time you're pregnant, it has been drummed into your psyche, making it hard to feel okay about eating enough nutritious food for you and your baby. After your baby's birth, it can result in shame when you look in the mirror or step on the scale. Recently, it's become harder to identify diet culture because the word *diet* is out of fashion. Now you hear about "clean eating," "superfoods," and "bad" or "toxic" foods. But don't be fooled, the message is the same: your postpartum body is a problem, something you need to fix—pronto. Of course, if you're motivated to change your shape, more power to you; just don't do it because you were pressured by cultural messages. Fortunately, there are ways to counter that messaging.

Reject the pressure of diet culture. Make an effort to identify the messages coming at you from the media and from your own mind. They are selling you a false bill of goods. Get angry at them, if you have to, in order to fully reject them. Instead of a "weight watchers" support group, form a support group with other moms fighting the social pressure to diet.

Respect your body's hunger and fullness. Listen to the wisdom of your body. It knows what it needs to keep you (and your baby) nourished. If your body says it's hungry, feed it. And let it tell you what it wants to eat. Listen when it tells you it's full. If you're in the habit of listening to the messages of diet culture, you may need some time to retrain yourself to these more intuitive messages. At first, you might not hear some of them. But no worries—a few mistakes won't make you unhealthy. Keep practicing this form of "mindful eating" and work toward a gradual but lasting shift in your attitudes toward food.

You're Feeling Over-Touched

Touch is a beautiful thing. Mark wasn't saying anything inherently wrong when he told Iris touch was his language of love and that he needed it. But sometimes we can have too much of a good thing. New moms, especially those who are breastfeeding, can become what's known as *over-touched*, or *touched out*. With your baby (and children) constantly touching your body, your skin wants to scream, "Stop!" Add to that your partner touching you to reignite intimacy, and you can become one touched-out mama.

It's not just the constant physical touch that creates the overwhelm, it's your baby's neediness that accompanies it. Newborns are completely dependent, and parents (especially breastfeeding moms) are on call 24/7. You don't have any down time when you can completely check out. As soon as your baby starts whimpering, you're needed. The never-ending demand creates a cumulative effect, similar to sleep deprivation, such that the last thing you want from your partner is to feel needed in any way. That is the case even if your need as a couple is for more connection and romance.

Here are two ways to help you overcome this.

Create new boundaries. Knowing you have some sovereignty over your physical and emotional space can go a long way toward healing the feeling of being touched out. I suggest making an agreement with your partner that lets you experience your own physical space for at least fifteen minutes every day, starting in early postpartum life. You could do this by leaving your home or by being alone in a room, or by any other way that works for you both. Breaking the tether from your baby and your partner for even a brief period daily can help heal the sense of too much touch, and it can also be preventive.

Balance touch with talk. A new stay-at-home mom I know recently told me about her experience of being touched out. If her partner wanted to touch her when he came home, she recoiled from what she felt was his need for her. However, they discovered that if she could first talk about her day and fill him in on everything, while he provided a good sounding board, that helped them as a couple heal her sense of being over-touched. One way to redefine romance when you're feeling touched out is to make an agreement that your partner will just be there for you when that is what you need most. You could agree to do this at a time of reunions (as we discussed in chapter 6) or at any other time that works for you both. Your partner could listen to you or hold you, or whatever you need, without having to receive something from you in return in that moment.

Conclusion

Reframing romance for life post–baby bomb is an ongoing adventure. It starts in pregnancy with hormonal and other physical changes but really hits full on after baby arrives. Successfully navigating these changes by redefining romance can give not only your sexuality but also your secure-functioning teamwork a new maturity and deepen your couple connection.

Another aspect of your partnership that may need a reboot is conflict resolution. Your time and energy to engage in conflict is clipped in a party of three, so it's helpful to find new tools to streamline your process for resolving disagreements. In the next chapter, we'll dig into ways to repair any hurt you've caused each other and to achieve win-wins.

CHAPTER 9

Fighting Fair

"Hey, Carmen, we gotta talk," Vince says as he walks down the stairs, carrying their infant daughter, Luna.

"Sure," Carmen says, pulling a piping hot cake out of the oven. It's the first time she's had the energy to bake since giving birth. However, juggling baby and cake turned out to be harder than she expected, and she had to enlist Vince's help with childcare. "I just need to see if this bad boy's ready. Gimme a sec. You're going to love this cake, Vince."

"I'm not in the mood for cake."

"How can you not be in the mood for cake? Everybody loves cake." Carmen leaves the cake on the counter and walks over to Vince, but her eyes are on Luna. "You're gonna love this cake," she coos.

"I said we need to talk," Vince says, his voice full of frustration.

"What's up?" Carmen says curtly as she grabs Luna, sits down, undoes her shirt, and brings the baby to her nipple.

"You said you'd watch Luna so I could brainstorm project ideas with Willis. Then, fifteen minutes into it, you interrupted and gave me Luna so you could finish your cake."

"Yeah, so I wouldn't injure her while I was baking. And the problem is?"

Vince glares at Carmen. *How can you not see the problem?* he thinks. "The problem," he says, voice rising, "is it was embarrassing to book that call and then have to suddenly cancel because I had Luna."

Hearing Vince's voice rise, Carmen feels an instinctive need to defend herself. "Let me get this straight. You're upset because I baked you a cake?"

"No!" Vince practically screams. "I'm upset because you broke the agreement we had that you'd watch Luna while I was on that call!"

Carmen shifts Luna to her other breast as she tries to remember that agreement. *Why should I feel guilty about asking for help,* she thinks, *when he agreed to take more responsibility for childcare?* "I don't understand," she says. "I watch Luna all day every day, and then I ask you to be a father ... and now it's a problem?"

"That's BS! You don't watch Luna all day every day!" Vince punctuates his words by pounding his right hand into the palm of his left hand. "Besides, you're missing the point. I arranged this call around your schedule, and then you decided to bake a cake and broke our agreement."

Luna starts to fuss. "Now you've upset the baby," Carmen snaps. "Just chill! I get interrupted on work calls all the time when she needs to eat. Yesterday I was on a call with the gallery, and you couldn't soothe her, so I had to nurse her as I finished my call."

"Like I have breasts? You hadn't pumped any milk, so what was I to do?"

"Figure it out, Vince! I'm just saying you're not the only one making sacrifices."

Vince throws up his hands in frustration. "I thought I could talk to you, but I guess I was wrong."

"I guess I was wrong thinking you could parent fifty-fifty with me!"

With that, Vince storms out of the house, without saying goodbye. Carmen feels her heart beating quickly and her breathing shallow. She is angry, tired, and confused. *What just happened?* she thinks. *I broke an agreement? What have I agreed to? All the childcare?*

♥♥♥

Conflict, fights, and disagreements are relatively common experiences in long-term partnerships. You have two different, complex, human (read: not perfect) people with two unique yet equally important perspectives, who're trying to live harmoniously together. What's more, they each come from a first-family upbringing that gave them deeply embedded ideas about the right and wrong ways to live. And then you bring a baby onto the scene. What could possibly go awry? With all this potential kindling, it's no wonder many conversations go haywire, catch fire, and become fights.

It might surprise you to hear me say that fighting per se is not a bad thing. In fact, there is bad fighting, and there is good fighting. Bad fighting is the kind Carmen and Vince typify: hurtful, frustrating battles that lead to nowhere but further fights. Good fighting is fair; it puts your disagreements on the table and lets you and your partner resolve them together in a manner that brings more peace, greater collaboration, and a deeper sense of secure functioning into your partnership.

In this chapter, you will learn how to become full-apology experts so your partner feels seen and understood, and their confidence in the relationship is restored. You will learn to repair hurts before they do permanent damage. I also break down what "fighting for two winners" means and how to find dual-winner resolution step by step.

Guiding Principle 9: You and your partner fight for two winners.

What started out as a bid by Vince for an apology from Carmen quickly escalated into a full-tilt fight. What Carmen didn't realize is that part of the principle of fighting for two winners is attending to the hurt partner first and foremost. There is a psychobiological reason for this. When a partner is hurt, alarm bells go off in their head, signaling the presence of imminent threat. That threat level needs to be reduced before any progress can be made. She also didn't realize that the solution wasn't either-or; it wasn't a choice between her baking a cake and Vince talking with his colleague.

In *Wired for Love*, Stan describes two parts of the brain: the warring brain and the loving brain. The warring parts of the brain (e.g., our amygdala, hypothalamus, and dorsal motor vagal complex), where our alarm bells live, he calls the "primitives." To turn off those alarm bells and engage peacefully so we can achieve win-win solutions, we need to activate what he calls the "ambassadors" (e.g., our hippocampus, ventral vagal complex, insula, and prefrontal cortex). You can think of these respective parts of your brain as your lower and higher natures. Your primitives operate on instinct, out of fear and self-preservation; they are more concerned with being the sole winner than finding a win-win. Their job is to keep you safe, not to build safe relationships. In contrast, your ambassadors are both rational and socially oriented; they have the ability to empathize and be cool tempered, as well as to find logical and equitable solutions. Your ambassadors know how to get you out of the messes your primitives get you into.

You and your partner must learn to engage your ambassadors if you want to become experts at fighting fair. With the help of your ambassadors, you must quickly heal any hurts, and then you must bargain a resolution that creates two winners. These two ambassador-driven skill sets are a total relationship Rx.

The first provides relief, repair, and understanding. The second ensures that you both feel satisfied, appreciated, and empowered—as individuals and as a couple. Let's look at each of these more closely.

Healing the Hurt

Inevitably, you are going to hurt your partner's feelings. And your partner will hurt yours. This can be a disaster—as it was for Carmen and Vince—or it can be a natural part of learning and loving. I'm not saying this to give you a free pass to go out and be a jerk to your partner; rather, I'm saying that the more comfort you can develop with your ability to make mistakes and learn from them, the easier it will be for you to make thoughtful and healing repairs in your partnership.

Let's look at how things went wrong for Carmen and Vince. When he was making a bid for repair, her primitives rose to the fore. Her responses were defensive and lacked accountability. For example, when he said he wasn't in the mood for cake (because they needed to talk), her instinctive response was "Everybody loves cake." She was defending herself rather than trying to listen to Vince. "What's the problem?" was her mantra each time he tried to express his feelings. Rather than bringing her ambassadors online, she let her primitives stay in charge. And they did what primitives would do in that situation: they changed the subject and avoided admitting any way in which she might have hurt Vince.

Many of us have never learned how to properly repair so that emotional injuries are healed and forgiven, not left to fester in a way that cracks our sense of security. If no one in your home offered real repair when you were growing up, how could you know how to offer that to a partner now? In my childhood, repair was offered but it sounded like, "I'm sorry you're hurt … but I needed to yell at you because you weren't listening." The reason for hurting someone was the highlighted part. As a result, relief and healing didn't follow. In addition, when we are tired, depleted, or running low on resources (think baby bomb), it's easier to make mistakes that can hurt each other. I'm going to show you instead how to lean on your ambassadors so you can let down your guard and understand how you hurt your partner, and then use this healing to build trust and security between you.

Here's a heal-the-hurt cheat sheet with the five things to remember when your partner says that their feelings are hurt or that they're uncomfortable with something you did or said.

Quick repair. Time is of the essence when it comes to healing the hurt. Waiting allows the primitives to dig in and makes it harder for the ambassadors to engage. The longer you wait, the more the hurt solidifies in long-term memory and the more difficult it will be to repair. So seize the moment and do a quick repair with your partner.

No distractions. Put down whatever you're working on or turn off the television; clear the deck so you can put your full attention on your partner. This signals to your partner how important they are to you, which is the beginning of the repair.

Offer a full apology. Just saying you're sorry isn't enough. You have to be sincere and take responsibility. A full apology takes ownership for whatever you did that caused the hurt, whether or not—and this is the key—you did it intentionally. Because rarely do partners intentionally hurt one another. Here are some examples of apology dos and don'ts.

Dos	Don'ts
"I'm sorry."	"I'm sorry, but ..."
"I'm sorry I said that."	"I'm sorry you felt that way."
"I believe you."	"That's your perspective, but ..."
"My behavior hurt you."	"I didn't mean it that way."
"I know I hurt you, and I'm sorry."	"If I hurt you, I'm sorry."
"I'm going to work on changing my behavior."	"You're too sensitive."

Engage in active listening. It's your job to listen so you can learn and understand how your behavior affected your partner. The "active" part of listening involves reflecting back what you heard your partner say. This allows (1) you to confirm that you heard accurately—or to correct what you reflect back, if it turns out you didn't hear correctly—and (2) your partner to have the experience of feeling heard and valued.

Talk face to face, eye to eye. You want to bust out your best sherlocking skills so you can fully take in your partner. And you want them to be able to see you clearly as well. (If you must offer a repair on the phone, that's okay, but you'll have to provide more verbal assurances, because your partner won't be able to see and read your face.) Watch not only for their pain but also for signs of relief. If you're tending to your partner, you should be able to see them physically soften. That's your cue that the repair is working. If this isn't the case, say so. For example, "I can see this isn't working. What am I not understanding? Do you know what would work?"

Revisiting Carmen and Vince

Let's see how—leading with her ambassadors and armed with an understanding about the dos and don'ts for an effective apology—Carmen might handle her conversation with Vince differently.

"Hey Carmen, can we talk?" Vince asks as he steps into the kitchen, carrying Luna.

Carmen looks up from pulling her cake out of the oven and sees Vince. His face is flushed. Immediately she puts the cake down and moves toward him. "You look upset, love. Is anything wrong?"

"Yeah, I'm really ticked off and hurt."

"Okay. I can see that. Let me take Luna and feed her so she won't fuss while we talk."

Vince feels his body relax a little. "Thanks. I feel better just hearing you say that."

"You're important to me, and I can tell you're upset." Carmen sits down on one of the kitchen counter barstools and puts Luna to her breast, then turns to Vince, her eyes gentle and curious. "Okay, tell me what's going on."

Vince leans on the counter and strokes the baby's head as he talks to Carmen. "You said you'd watch Luna so I could brainstorm with Willis, and then you came up and handed me Luna when I was only fifteen minutes into my call. You broke our agreement. That's why I'm hurt."

Carmen wants to make sure she understood, so she asks, "You're upset because I broke our agreement about who was watching Luna. Is that right?"

"Yeah. It was embarrassing to have to cancel my call with Willis, especially when I'm the one who scheduled it in the first place."

Carmen pauses to process what Vince said. She feels a flash of annoyance that it wasn't easy just to bake her cake. She also notices feeling shame over making a mistake. But then she makes a conscious effort to shift her focus to Vince's experience. "I can see how my behavior frustrated you," she says after a minute. "I didn't think about our agreement when I brought Luna up to you. I'm sorry. It slipped my mind that you were on with Willis; I was only thinking about my cake. Sorry, love."

"Yeah. It wasn't cool, Carmen."

"It wasn't. I agree."

Vince feels his body relax more and his breathing begin to deepen.

Carmen notices this too and leans toward him, saying one more time, "I'm sorry, babe. It won't happen again. Our agreements are important to both of us, and I need to do better at remembering them!"

Vince laughs. "I'm sure getting more sleep would help you remember. I know you're more tired and more forgetful than usual. I appreciate your apology. Thanks."

♥♥♥

We see here that Carmen made an effort to do a quick repair with Vince. Not allowing time for his hurt feelings to fester and for their respective primitives to take over made a huge difference in their interaction. Their disagreement didn't escalate, and they were able to stay connected and tend to their bond. Of course, an apology is not going to permanently heal all the hurt in a relationship. The next step in fighting fair is to negotiate around the situation in which the hurt arose. For Carmen and Vince, that will involve examining the agreement that was broken.

What Your Kids Should See

Carmen mentioned she would nurse Luna while the couple talked. Before we move on, I'd like to highlight this, because it raises an important point: how you and your partner handle fights becomes the model your kids will carry into life. When Charlie and I find things getting tense between us, and Jude is there, we stop and schedule time to talk later. Then we tell Jude what's going on. Usually it's along the lines of "We're trying to figure something out, and we haven't cracked the code yet. But we will. And we're okay. You don't have to worry about us loving and caring for each other." Sometimes finding a time without your child present isn't possible. And that's fine, as long as your ambassadors remain in charge. The message you want your kids to get is "My parents may fight, but they do it fairly, without hurting each other, and it doesn't mean they don't love each other or love me."

What you don't want is your kids witnessing a fight run by your primitives. First off, I should clarify that any form of physical violence—such as slapping, biting, pushing, hitting, throwing things—is scary and potentially traumatic to kids. This discussion is about fighting fair, so in this context, I'm not even going to consider physical violence "fighting." It's abuse, and it's unacceptable. If physical violence happens in your family even one time, you need to seek outside help. But that's not to say that—short of violence—your primitives will never take over a fight. Your (and your partner's) primitives may yell or scream or swear or say things you don't mean. What if that happens, and you can't stop yourselves? Here are some strategies for getting back into ambassador territory:

- Immediately repair with each other, using the principles of healing the hurt we've discussed.

- Also repair with your child (as I described doing with Jude). As your child matures, you may want to ask about their feelings after witnessing a fight, so they have a chance to share and hold you accountable for how your behavior affected them.

- You can even repair with your baby. When I changed Jude's diaper, I used to narrate, "I'm going to take off your diaper now. This is me lifting up your legs …" I found it helped. You might think infants can't understand if you say, "Your parents are trying to figure something out," but I really believe they can!

- Agree with your partner to set boundaries for your fights. Having this agreement will increase your awareness in any fights going forward.

- Establish a safe word you and your partner can use to signal each other if you are fighting in front of your child in a way that crosses that boundary.

Your Vulnerabilities

In *Wired for Love*, Stan postulates that we all have three or four vulnerabilities that hound us through life. If you thought you had hundreds, hearing it's likely the same few repeat offenders may come as good news. These vulnerabilities serve as triggers and set off your alarm bells. To quickly repair when a fight occurs, it is helpful to know what your alarm bells are. This isn't to say it **will** always be those habitual vulnerabilities and nothing else. In fact, post–baby bomb, certain vulnerabilities may stand out more than others. Here are some examples:

- Feeling unfairly burdened. ("It's always me doing the pickups *and* the drop-offs.")

- Feeling unheard. ("I feel like it doesn't matter if I say I think potty training would work better this way.")

- Feeling blamed or criticized. ("I'm always the bad-cop parent." "Baby has a diaper blowout, and *I* put the diaper on wrong; it's always *my* fault.")

- Fear of being out of control. ("I'm afraid I won't know how to take care of a newborn." "With all the demands of parenthood, I'll never get what *I* need.")

- Fear of being unloved or forgotten. ("I'm afraid my partner won't find me sexy anymore." "My partner is always with the baby; there's no time left for me.")

- Fear of being alone. ("My relationships never last; I'll end up a single parent.")

Know Your Alarm Bells

In this exercise, you will identify the alarm bells that ring most loudly in your relationship. I suggest you first do this alone, then compare notes with your partner.

Listen for your alarm bells. Find a quiet time and place for self-reflection. If you like, you can do a short meditation to get you into an introspective mood.

Now review some of the conflicts you and your partner have had or some of the times you were angry with or hurt by your partner. What's key here is to let your ambassadors run this exercise. How do you know if you're doing that? Your ambassadors are able to look objectively at what happened, without getting emotionally embroiled. If you find yourself "getting back into" the heated emotion of a fight, that's your primitives rising up.

For each fight or angry incident you review, ask your ambassadors, "What were my alarm bells there?" Look for patterns and consider the vulnerabilities named above. Are you able to notice a theme?

Journal about your alarm bells. As you reflect on your alarm bells, take the help of your journal. Compare the reactions you had in different conflict situations and see if you can cull and combine them to identify the main ones. Remember, most of us only have a handful of vulnerabilities that crop up repeatedly.

Make sure your vulnerabilities are statements about *you*, not about your partner. You aren't asking "What set off my alarm bells?" For example:

- Correct: "I feel like I'm to blame for everything." "I tend to feel like everything is my fault."

- Incorrect: "I overreact whenever you blame me." "You make me feel like I'm at fault."

Get with your partner. You want to do this at a peaceful time, free of fighting, after you have each individually identified your respective alarm bells. Sit down together and share your three or four main alarm bells. Make sure it's your ambassadors doing the talking, and not your primitives reengaging in a conflict.

Unless your partner gives you explicit permission to do so, avoid pointing out what you see as their alarm bells. Instead, concentrate on listening.

Finally, discuss how you might use this new information during future conflict situations. For example, you might agree to monitor your alarm bells during arguments. Or you might agree on a signal you can give when your ambassadors notice alarm bells going off.

Fighting for Two Winners

As we have discussed, the ability to create win-win solutions is a hallmark of secure-functioning partner teams. Both partners' ambassadors light the way as they continue to go back and forth, negotiating until they find their mutual happy spot.

Sometimes you'll hear a win-win equated with a compromise, and sometimes you'll hear them presented as mutually exclusive strategies. Let me explain how I'm using the terms here. In a compromise, each partner gives up something for the sake of the greater good of their coupledom. In this sense, compromise can be seen as emphasizing what you each give up. In contrast, a win-win focuses on what you both gain. You both acknowledge that neither of your individual solutions is fully satisfactory to both, so you come up with a third option.

Despite this distinction, I think a compromise can be part of a win-win solution. As you negotiate, you can include some element of compromise—something you trade off with each other. For example, Charlie and I might decide he will watch Jude so I can go for a run, and when I get home, I'll watch Jude so Charlie can work on some photographs. To a win-win purist, that might not be considered legit, but in the context of secure functioning—where your mandate is to take care of each other even if it means sacrificing something you want so your partner gets what they want—I think it works.

You know you've reached a win-win when both you and your partner can high-five at the solution, confident neither of you will feel resentful, cheated, or bitter about it. The following are guidelines for negotiating win-wins.

Operate from your ambassadors. Don't let your primitives run the show. Don't even give them a seat at the table. Both you and your partner will need your creative problem-solving abilities and your empathy fully online to reach a win-win. If any of your primitives hijack the bargaining, stop immediately and tend to that. You need all your ambassadors online for this to work.

In *Wired for Love*, Stan encourages couples to wave a "friendly flag" during a disagreement to keep your primitives from feeling threatened. Friendly flags are anything that signals to your partner that you're a team and in this together: saying, "I know we'll find our win-win" or "I'm glad we're collaborating on this," or giving a nonverbal sign, such as a smile.

Name the problem. First things first, you want to make sure you're both trying to solve the same problem. In our original scenario, Carmen and Vince never got to first base with that. After you've defined what's not working, discuss any attempts you've made collectively or individually to solve it.

Take turns spitballing ideas. Maintain a safe environment in which you're allowed to put any ideas on the table for consideration. When you feel safe, it's easier to get your creative juices flowing. Think outside the box. What could you each contribute to make a solution work? Each idea is entitled to an open and fair discussion to determine if it could be a win for both partners.

Equal veto power. Narrow down your ideas by eliminating those that aren't wins for both of you. If one of you says no, that's a nix. You must both dismiss the idea. Trying to repackage an idea that was dismissed and submitting it for another round of spitballing can upend the negotiation if one partner doesn't feel their no was respected. Instead, it can help if a partner who says no also offers an alternative solution. That will make it harder for one partner to keep a heavy foot on the veto pedal.

Hone in on your win-win. The goal is for both you and your partner to feel positive about the resolution. When both of you are feeling good (or at least 80 percent good), you've done it! If you can't find a win-win during your initial attempt, don't sweat it. Put it down for now, and circle back to it later.

Revisiting Carmen and Vince's Negotiation

Let's see how it went when Carmen and Vince sat down later that day to negotiate a win-win. They began by naming the problem as Carmen's fatigue, because, as Vince put it, "It's not like you to space on one of our agreements." Note that another couple in a similar situation might name a different problem, such as the need to shore up how they finalize agreements or the need to support each other when they feel frazzled.

"Maybe one way to address your fatigue," Vince says, "is for me to start doing night duty so you can sleep."

"That's sweet, babe," Carmen says. "And I am bone tired some days. But honestly, the hardest thing is not getting downtime. Being tethered to Luna is what's wearing me out. And it bugs me when you can't soothe her, so you bring her to me to nurse when I thought I was maybe getting some downtime."

"Okay," says Vince thoughtfully. "Sounds like this might be more about your feeling that our responsibilities aren't equitable, and less about just fatigue?"

Carmen nods. "For the purpose of finding a win-win, let's rename the problem as an inequity in our roles." Then she hesitates. "You know I love nursing Luna. I love being a mom. Is it silly for me to complain ...?"

Vince immediately jumps in to reassure her. "It's not silly at all. I can see how being tethered to Luna for the past four months has worn you out and that it's not fair I don't carry the same tether. Am I understanding you correctly?"

"You are," Carmen says, then adds, "but I'm not going to quit breastfeeding, so don't even suggest that as part of a win-win."

Vince laughs. "I won't go there. But what about pumping more?"

Carmen groans. "Pumping's a drag. And especially having to clean up all the parts afterward." She stops abruptly. "Hey! Here's an idea: what if you started washing my pump parts?"

"I could absolutely do that!" Vince is about to high-five Carmen, but he holds off and says, "What else could help it be more fair?"

She has a quick answer: "Being able to get out of the house untethered a few times a week."

"So you'd pump a bottle, then I'd wash the parts. And I'd have that bottle on hand while you're off footloose and fancy free?"

Carmen grins. "Now you're talking!"

Vince grins back, happy they're zeroing in on a win-win. But he has another proposal to thrown into the mix. "Can you do something for me?"

"What?"

"Will you consider sleeping on the couch and letting me do night duty at least once a week? I know you're afraid your milk supply will go down, but I'd really like to support you getting more rest. You said you're bone tired. That's not good, babe."

Carmen agrees to consider that. "I don't want to sleep on the couch, but I think you're right that a night off would help me. How about I pump a bottle now and head out for hike so I can think about it?"

"That's a win-win."

♥♥♥

Vince and Carmen did a great job listening to each other, clarifying the problem, and exploring what would and wouldn't work. At first, it might seem that Vince is making more sacrifices than Carmen, that he's coming away with less of a "what's in it for me." But that's not the case; he's driven by the guiding principles that say the couple comes first and his partner is in his care. So when he asks Carmen to let him take on night duty—and frames it as "do something for me"—he means that literally. Carmen getting more rest will benefit him because it benefits her and their couple team.

These partners were able to find a win-win quite quickly. Not all win-wins are as smooth as in this redo, so if your first or second attempt is a bit more wonky or is hijacked by your own or your partner's primitives, don't give up. The more you practice this type of conflict resolution, the better you'll get at it.

Common Fights for Parents

Certain issues tend to come up frequently between partners with a baby bomb or two. It can be helpful to know what these are so you can look out for them.

- sleeping arrangements and interventions

- discipline

- what and how much to give your child

- what's safe and unsafe for your child

- nutrition and eating habits

- who else gets to care for your child

- childcare and household management equity

- television and screen time

In addition, as Stan reminds us—most recently in a *New York Times* article that quoted his remarks about fighting during the pandemic—it's helpful to know that most couples' fighting centers on five broad topics: sex, mess, kids (just discussed), money, and time. Often these fights are fueled by each partner's first-family issues. For example, if your parents fought about money, chances are you'll be supercharged in disagreements with your partner about how to spend and save money. Or you may try to avoid the topic altogether in an effort not to follow in your parents' footsteps. Either way, naming these common and often-heated topics can help you and your partner approach them with an awareness of their heat.

RENEGOTIATING WIN-WIN AGREEMENTS

As you practice becoming more adept at reaching win-wins, it can be useful to return to your foundational couple agreements. In chapter 3, we talked about keeping that agreement alive through revisions and updates, as well as making the tending of your agreements a daily practice. Conflicts in your relationship can serve as a sign that an agreement needs tweaking. This exercise gives you an opportunity to assess this.

1. Take an inventory of any recent (or current) conflicts or areas of friction in your relationship. You can do this on your own or together with your partner. The list can be short or long.

2. Go through the list and identify any conflicts that relate to an agreement between you and your partner. If none relate to an agreement, identify a conflict you feel could benefit from an agreement.

3. Now get with your partner and decide if you both want to renegotiate the agreement related to this conflict (or negotiate a new agreement if there is no existing agreement).

4. Follow the process and principles discussed in this chapter to achieve a win-win agreement that addresses your point of conflict.

What Makes This Principle Hard?

Fighting with your partner is rarely—two-blue-moons-in-a-year rarely—easy for anyone. It's especially challenging if you're living largely on the red or blue part of the attachment continuum. If your parents offered you full repair when they hurt you, troubleshot to find win-wins with you, and put your relationship with them first, then you will most likely act with security in your partnership. As a yellow person, you may not like conflict, but you can handle being in the thick of it. However, if you didn't experience fighting fairly in your first family, then you're more likely to struggle with conflict now. Let's look at how blues and reds—either you or your partner, or both—deal with conflict and at some of the skills you can learn to fight fair even if your parents didn't model them for you.

Blues Fighting Fair

Hey, blue, I see you! If you're blue, you most likely prefer to avoid conflict. You're probably not the first one in your relationship to mention any problems. When your partner does something annoying, you may withdraw so you can be alone and calm down. You can also withdraw emotionally, without explanation. You may dismiss or minimize any comments you fear could lead to a fight. Because you believe you are solely responsible for taking care of yourself, you may feel confused or frustrated when your partner wants to work through a disagreement with you. This is what blues can do about conflicts.

If you're a blue:

- Take a time-out before you get overwhelmed. A time-out is not the same as withdrawing; it's out in the open and purposeful. Tell your partner you need alone time (be explicit about how long), grab a hug if you can, and then go and regroup.

- If your partner criticizes you, remind yourself they're criticizing your behavior, not you. Even if you did something wrong, that doesn't make you a bad person.

- Develop a mantra for support. For example: "My job isn't to *be* right; it's to *get* this right." "I can feel upset and still be okay." "We still love each other even if we're arguing." "I have nothing to be ashamed of."

If your partner is a blue:

- If you see your partner getting overwhelmed, suggest a brief break to regroup. "Let's do a time-out. I'll watch the baby if you want to take a walk. How about we talk again this evening?"

- Knowing your partner is sensitive to criticism, use language that calls out behavior not character. For example: "I get upset when you leave without letting me know where you're going or when you'll return."

Reds Fighting Fair

Hey red! You're a high-drama fighter; you like to turn up the heat when disagreeing. To keep it hot, you may bring up multiple topics at once, which can be overwhelming to your partner. Also, you may go on tangents when speaking because talking calms you down when you're upset. You want things to be fair, but you worry they won't be if you don't keep score. In fact, you may be secretly afraid of finding a resolution; deep down, you fear a resolution won't work, so it's better to keep fighting. The following is what reds can do about conflict.

If you're a red:

- Stay with one issue until you and your partner find a resolution for that, before bringing up another issue.

- If you feel criticized, pause before responding. Ask your partner for help. For example: "I need a friendly flag to be able to do this together." Or invoke your own mantra, such as "I'm loveable and worthy of belonging. We'll figure this out."

- If you become aware of yourself getting agitated as you and your partner hone in on a win-win, congratulate yourself on your awareness. Use it to help yourself get across the finish line. Since it helps you to talk things out when you're upset, talk about all the ways your win-win will work.

If your partner is a red

- Use active listening to help your partner stay on track. "You said you were upset that I got home late last night. So I'm confused why we're talking about who cleans the bathroom. I want to address the hurt I caused by being late first."

- Offer reassurance that you guys will get through this in one piece, by saying things like "I love you, and we'll find a way" and by offering nonverbal support (hugs, smiles, and moving in closer).

Conclusion

Hopefully I've convinced you that if you and your partner learn to let your ambassadors take the lead, fighting can be a natural part of your relationship and can even lead to growth. In a secure-functioning relationship, partners don't let hurts fester; they know how to quickly heal any hurt and then move on to find a win-win solution that takes their partnership to a higher level. Which brings us to the final chapter, in which we talk about how you pull all the guiding principles together as you solidify your future as a couple.

CHAPTER 10

Looking Ahead

Sasha and her wife, Kerry, are in the bathroom getting ready for bed, while Chloé sleeps in her bassinet.

"There's something I want to do tomorrow," Sasha says.

Kerry reaches for the floss as she hazards a guess: "Pick up more diapers?"

"I'm on it with the diapers. Like we agreed: I buy them, you change 'em. Next week we switch off." Sasha smiles, proud of their win-win. "But, no, actually, this is more long term. I want to call the adoption agency."

Kerry stops flossing mid-stroke. "What?"

"The adoption agency," Sasha repeats. "I want to call them and get the ball rolling. It took four years to find Chloé. We can't afford to wait if we want our kids close in age."

Kerry didn't see this coming—certainly not now, with Chloé only a few months old. "I'm still torn up by what we went through, all the times we thought we were getting a baby only to have the rug pulled out from under us." She sits down on the edge of the tub and stares at the floor, the familiar mix of sadness and anxiety rising within her. "I don't know if I can do it all over again."

Sasha can see from Kerry's tells how disturbed she is, but her own heart is aching so much for another child that she charges ahead anyway. "Don't say that! I've always said how much I love big families. And you never objected. Not once. So, my warrior wife, you just have to toughen up a bit."

Kerry doesn't say anything.

As Sasha watches the tears stream down Kerry's face, she worries she's pushing too hard. "I can see you're hurting. I'm sorry," she says, reaching out her hand. "Come, let's go to bed. We can keep talking tomorrow."

But Kerry pulls away. "You go on. I need some space." She gets up, brushes by Sasha and stops at the bathroom door, then turns back to say, "And I *don't* want to toughen up! I don't want to do any of that again. I just want to enjoy Chloé, our perfect little angel, and leave it at that."

Sasha doesn't follow her. *You need space to heal?* she thinks. *Well, so do I! But we have to move forward. If I get the process started, I know you'll thank me later on.*

♥♥♥

Deciding whether or not to have another child—let alone when to begin trying—is a big decision for most couples post–baby bomb. Add the heartache of a long, tumultuous adoption process or IVF journey or of a pregnancy loss, and it can be even more difficult. In moments like these, partners need to bust out all the guiding principles and put them into practice to tend to their secure-functioning team.

This chapter presents the final guiding principle, which is both a summation of the previous nine principles and the glue that holds those principles together. It's like the steady hand that guides you through all the choppy waters you two will encounter. If you remember to follow this principle, you'll have what it takes to find your way out of any jam, no matter what! In this chapter, you will also learn how to futurize so you and your partner can set family goals and realize your dreams as you look ahead.

Guiding Principle 10: You and your partner parent and partner with sensitivity, respect, and trust.

A secure-functioning relationship is designed for the long haul, to give you and your partner the best possible chance at finding a love that is lasting and sustainable. The nine principles we've covered give you a solid team—two people who know how to take care of each other and your family, make agreements and decisions, value needs, coregulate, achieve balance, keep romance alive, and create win-wins. If you adhere to these principles, they will carry you into the future you want to live. Can you count on that? Yes, you can ... but not without also adhering to the three partnership qualities at the core of each principle: sensitivity, respect, and trust.

Because sensitivity, respect, and trust are baked into the other principles, they're mentioned throughout the book; here I highlight them. These three ingredients are your not-so-secret sauce. Without them shining brightly in all your interactions, any of the principles can fall short. For example, Sasha and Kerry show some fluency with sherlocking, they know about win-wins, and Sasha is at least familiar with apologies. Even so, their interaction implodes due to a glaring lack of sensitivity, respect, and trust. Before we break each down into bite-size pieces so you can consider how to implement it, here are some examples of how they might sound.

- Sensitivity. "I see your pain. Tell me how I can support you." "I know how much you want this. Let me help." "I see that look in your eye. Am I right?"

- Respect. "I want to understand why you feel that way." "I don't think I could do that, but it's so great you can." "I didn't think of that; thank you for bringing it up."

- Trust. "I know you'll always be there for me and the baby." "I won't let you down." "My care is in your hands."

Sensitivity

Sensitivity is, by definition, the ability to sense slight impressions and to care about them. This comes into play in secure-functioning relationships in a number of ways. Perhaps the most obvious is the practice of sherlocking, which is based on your ability to be sensitive to your partner in any given moment. You have to be alert to slight changes in your partner in order to recognize their tells and respond in a way that shows you care.

Sensitivity can also be seen as the basis of respect. For example, if Sasha had been sensitive in that moment, she would have immediately noticed Kerry's signs of distress. She would have then shown respect for Kerry's feelings and continued to use her sensitivity to monitor how Kerry was reacting to their discussion.

Traditional mainstream culture assumes that sensitivity is gender related and belongs more to women than to men. However, there is no psychobiological reason for that belief. In fact, a secure-functioning relationship relies on both partners' ability to treat each other with sensitivity.

Respect

We all long to be respected and believed. We want our partner to affirm our experience before asserting their own. Sasha showed no respect for Kerry's experience when she told her to "toughen up" instead of legitimizing her feelings. You may not feel the same way or agree with your partner at all times. In fact, you probably won't! But you need to show respect for them at all times.

We've already talked about respect in the context of the other guiding principles. For example, we talked about valuing and respecting each other's needs, respecting your couple agreements, and treating each other with respect when you make decisions or negotiate a win-win. In these and other contexts, you show respect by practicing active listening, being curious, and yielding to your partner's experience. You set your position aside so you can really listen and understand where they're coming from. Don't jump in and tell them why they're wrong and you're right; that's not respectful. Of course, you may need to speak up to help them better understand your perspective, but first try to understand and respect theirs.

Keep in mind that respect isn't selfless. It benefits both of you. When your partner feels respected, their nervous system is relaxed, and they can partner better than when their nervous system is buzzing because they feel disrespected.

Trust

Trust is the abiding confidence that you can feel safe and secure with your partner—now and always. It's both something you earn and something you give. Trust is based on respect, and you and your partner build trust with each other one small act of respect at a time. On the flipside, each time you neglect your partner, say something cruel, or share something private with an outsider, you undermine trust. When Sasha barreled ahead even though she saw Kerry hurting, she broke her trust. No wonder Kerry wasn't ready to accept an apology; she didn't trust that Sasha really meant it or that she (Kerry) would be safe if they continued talking. If Sasha goes ahead with calling the adoption agency on her own, she will further break her trust.

Trust is inherent in the other nine guiding principles. For example, putting your coupledom first and agreeing to take care of each other require a foundation of trust. You have to trust that your partner will treat you as an insider. You have to trust that when you show vulnerability and express your needs, your partner will be there for you. And this trust must be reciprocal. Just as you fully trust your partner to care for you, see you, and help you, your partner must have the same degree of trust in you. Consider making an agreement that spells out what trust will look like in your relationship and how you will handle any breaches of trust.

Going for Your Big Dreams

So far, we've looked at the ten guiding principles as something to learn now, as you await your baby bomb, or as something to integrate into your current life with baby. But your baby bomb is only the beginning. Life continues over the years, sometimes with challenges coming at you from all sides. Yes, you'll have the guiding principles to help you meet those challenges, but it's also helpful to have a specific practice that sets you on a path to realizing your dreams going forward. Futurizing is that practice. I introduced you to futurizing in chapter 4, where you used it to imagine how a decision might play out. Here you will use it to set long-term goals, to create the family you want. Let's see how Sasha and Kerry use their take two to futurize about expanding their family.

Revisiting Sasha and Kerry

Sasha and Kerry have finished watching a show, and it's not yet time to get ready for bed. After getting her wife's permission to talk about something on her mind, Sasha says, "I've been feeling we should start the process of getting Chloé a sibling. What do you think?"

Kerry looks surprised. "You mean now?"

"Soon, yeah. Before Chloé's much older."

Kerry is quiet, looking down at the rug.

"What's going on, hun?" Sasha says, "I can see you're upset."

Kerry nods, indicating that Sasha's assessment is true. "I just don't know if I want to go through that again," she says, her lower lip trembling. "We have Chloé, but my heart is still broken from all the other babies we weren't able to bring home."

Sasha moves closer to her wife and puts an arm around her. She gently wipes Kerry's tears and waits.

After a few minutes, Kerry says, "Thanks for understanding. That makes me feel better. And I do know how much you want another child."

"Yes," Sasha says, "but not if it's not feeling right for you now."

Kerry considers that for a minute. While she's always admired Sasha's passion for her dreams, she herself tends to be more open-ended about what she wants their life to look like. "How about if we futurize a bit?" she says. "I'm not as good at that as you are, and I can't promise my feelings will shift instantly, but I think it would help to do some goal setting around this."

Sasha welcomes the suggestion and offers to go first. "Here's what I see if we start contacting adoption agencies now. It'll take a couple years to find another child. By then, Chloé might be, say, three, and they'd still be close in age. Maybe we even start a third adoption. I see a bustling household, full of happy kids. And two happy moms."

When it's her turn, Kerry says, "I see us going through the next couple years facing one disappointment after another as we try to adopt again. I see myself getting to the point where I'm robbed of enjoying my time parenting Chloé." She pauses and sees Sasha looking at her with genuine curiosity, exuding encouragement, which helps her dip into a deeper vision. "If I look beyond all the disappointment, I see our home with a couple of kids. Maybe not close in age. Or … maybe we've adopted a couple older kids. That might be easier than adopting a baby." She stops and looks at Sasha and laughs. "Yeah, maybe we've adopted three teens, and it's the same bustling house you're imagining!"

"Wow," Sasha says. "I never really considered adopting older kids."

"Would you consider it?"

"I'm not sure," Sasha says. "But this futurizing has blown open a lot of options."

"It sounds like we might be working toward setting the goal of an expanded family," Kerry says. "Especially if I can get behind your dream of a full house, and you can get behind my idea of waiting to adopt again. We just need more time and more discussions about how to reach our goal. But this feels like a good start."

♥♥♥

You can see that this time Sasha was more attuned to Kerry; she was more sensitive and didn't push her agenda, but she also didn't deny her own desires. Feeling respected by Sasha, Kerry was able to move past her intense emotions and begin to envision their future—something she avoided doing before. Futurizing helped these two look ahead in new ways so that—whether they ultimately decide to expand their family now, later, or never—it will be because that is in line with the vision they created together for their future.

Futurizing

Use this exercise to set goals for your family in a way that allows you to be more proactive in shaping the direction your lives will take. You can do the first two steps individually if you prefer, but you will want to involve your partner as you progress so you can set goals together.

Pick what you want to futurize about. Your topic can be related to a general life direction (like looking into your family's crystal ball) or to a more specific issue (such as the size of your family, where you want to live, or sources of income).

Project into the future. Focusing on your chosen topic, think about what your lives might look like in the future. Ask yourself: If we follow this course, what will our life be like …

- in one year?
- in five years?
- in ten years?

Depending on your topic, you may want to adjust the time frames for greater relevance. If you are doing this step with your partner, take turns sharing what you futurize. Your future scenarios don't all have to be positive. It's okay if this exercise reveals some negative outcomes. You can use that information to guide your goal setting.

Set your goal(s). Even if you did the first steps by yourself, this is where you want to get with your partner. Go through your futurizing for the three time frames and compare your visions. Do you both see the same thing in one year, five years, ten years? Were you able to see that far into the future? In what ways are your visions similar or conflicting?

Take all your data and look for common ground. See if you can come up with a goal that matches your vision. Don't limit yourselves to looking at this task as just decision-making, as a choice between doing X or Y (as you did in chapter 4). Rather, use this opportunity to set long-range, big-picture goals for your family. It's your future; step up and create it!

What Makes These Principles Easy?

Yes, you read correctly! We've looked at lots of factors that might make things hard, but ultimately, this book is about creating a relationship that's easy. What makes it easy is your commitment to leaning in to all ten guiding principles and fully investing in your team of two. When you do this, you create a safe and secure relationship that feels like the home you've always wanted to live in.

You don't have to be yellow secure to do this. And you don't have to have had parents who did this either. The coolest thing about secure-functioning relationships is that anyone can learn how to do this. It's not about slaving away on your partnership to make it perfect; it's about tending to it daily, as you would a beloved garden. It's about learning more and more each day about how to love your partner while loving yourself.

Especially in recent months, it's felt as though the world has thrown multiple curveballs at Charlie and me and our family, leaving us reeling at moments. More than ever, we've had to draw on all ten guiding principles, reassess what we envisioned for ourselves, regroup, and look ahead in new ways. As we do this, the tarot card I'd use to describe my experience is the World card. For me, the World reflects our partnership coming full circle, coming together, finding deep joy and fulfillment even in the face of inescapable and unprecedented change. It sums up the journey of our coupledom, a journey I feel so fortunate to be on. You and your partner can journey the World card too. I'm truly excited for you both and for your baby bomb(s) to boot.

Acknowledgments

To my wonderful coauthor: Stan, thanks for teaching me and encouraging me to develop my gifts. You saw a couple therapist in me before I could.

Thank you to the most phenomenal editor, Jude Berman. We are the dream team. I'm so grateful. To TBT, thanks for believing in this project and cheerleading me on with your giant lioness heart.

A big thank you to all my magical helpers, who conspired to love, support, and guide me throughout this journey: Naomi Buckley, Ryan Heffington, Maximilla Lukacs, Dr. Clarissa Pinkola Estés, Roo Krout, Cynthia Ess, Allison Carter, Bryce Longton, KK Karnaky, Paula and Steve Chipman, Jim McGuire, Ann Bartelstein, Aurisha Smolarski, Jennye Garibaldi, Jessica Snow, Sarah Rodman-Alvarez, and Chynna Smith.

To my sister, Allison Headlee, you are my oldest and dearest friend. Your fierce love is unmatched. Thanks for a lifetime of love and support.

And finally, thanks to my mom and dad. Dad, you showed me the love of playing with words from the moment I baby bombed into your life. Mom, you taught me I could do anything I dreamed, "one step at a time." Thanks for the undying encouragement only a mother can offer.

Resources for Professional Help

Resources for perinatal mood disorders

Anxiety and Depression Association of America (ADAA): adaa.org/find-help-for/women/perinatalmooddisorders

Postpartum Support International (PSI): www.postpartum.net/get-help/locations

Postpartum Health Alliance: postpartumhealthalliance.org

Resources for couple therapy

Each of the following has a directory of couple therapists you can research and contact.

Stan Tatkin's PACT Institute: thepactinstitute.wildapricot.org

The Gottman Institute: www.gottman.com/couples/find-a-therapist

Sue Johnson's Emotionally Focused Therapy (EFT): iceeft.com/find-a-therapist

References

Ainsworth, Mary D. S. *Patterns of Attachment: A Psychological Study of the Strange Situation.* New York: Lawrence Erlbaum, 1978.

Bologna, Caroline. "23 Times Tina Fey Hilariously Summed Up Parenting." *HuffPost,* May 18, 2017. www.huffpost.com/entry/23-times-tina-fey -hilariously-summed-up-parenting_n_591a7d9de4b0809be15797ea.

Bowlby, John. *A Secure Base: Parent-Child Attachment and Healthy Human Development.* New York: Basic Books, 1988.

Cantarow, Ellen. "No Kids." *The Village Voice,* January 15, 1985.

Cowan, Carolyn Pape, and Philip A. Cowan. *When Partners Become Parents: The Big Life Change for Couples.* New York: Basic Books, 1992.

Chung, YoonKyung, Barbara Downs, Danielle H. Sandler, and Robert Sienkiewicz. *The Parental Gender Earnings Gap in the United States.* Washington DC: U.S. Census Bureau, Center for Economic Studies, 2017. www2.census.gov/ces/wp/2017/CES-WP-17-68.pdf.

Fisher, Helen E. "Brains Do It: Lust, Attraction, and Attachment." *Dana Foundation Cerebrum,* January 1, 2000. www.dana.org/article /brains-do-it-lust-attraction-and-attachment.

Karp, Harvey. *The Happiest Baby on the Block.* New York: Bantam, 2002.

LeMasters, E. E. "Parenthood as Crisis." *Marriage and Family Living,* 19 (1957): 352–55. doi.org/10.2307/347802.

Marche, Stephen. "How to End Pandemic Fights with Your Partner." *New York Times,* June 8, 2020. www.nytimes.com/2020/06/08/well /family/marriage-relationships-fighting-couples-quarantine.html.

Miller, Claire Cain. "Children Hurt Women's Earnings, but Not Men's (Even in Scandinavia)." *New York Times,* February 5, 2018. www .nytimes.com/2018/02/05/upshot/even-in-family-friendly-scandinavia -mothers-are-paid-less.html.

Nahman, Haley. "Esther Perel on Why Marriage After Kids Is So Hard (and How to Fix It)." *Man Repeller,* March 14, 2018. www.repeller.com /2018/03/marriage-after-kids-advice.html.

Obama, Michelle. *Becoming.* New York: Random House, 2018.

O'Malley, Deirdre, Agnes Higgins, Cecily Begley, Deirdre Daly, and Valerie Smith. "Prevalence of and Risk Factors Associated with Sexual Health Issues in Primiparous Women at 6 and 12 Months Postpartum: A Longitudinal Prospective Cohort Study (the MAMMI Study)." *BMC Pregnancy Childbirth* 18, no. 196 (2018). doi.org/10.1186/s12884-018-1838-6.

Richter, David, Michael D. Krämer, Nicole K. Y. Tang, Hawley E. Montgomery-Downs, and Sakari Lemola. "Long-Term Effects of Pregnancy and Childbirth on Sleep Satisfaction and Duration of First-Time and Experienced Mothers and Fathers. *Sleep* 42, no. 4 (2019). doi.org/10.1093/sleep/zsz015.

Riquin, Elise, Claire Lamas, Isabelle Nicolas, Corinne Dugre Lebigre, Florence Curt, Henri Cohen, Guillaume Legendre, Maurice Corcos, and Nathalie Godart. "A Key for Perinatal Depression Early Diagnosis: The Body Dissatisfaction." *Journal of Affective Disorders* 245 (2019): 340–347. doi.org/10.1016/j.jad.2018.11.032.

Sears, William. "New Parents' 8 Most-Asked Questions." *Parenting.* www.parenting.com/article/new-parents-8-most-asked-questions.

Shapiro, Alyson Fearnley, John M. Gottman, and Sybil Carrère. "The Baby and the Marriage: Identifying Factors that Buffer Against Decline in Marital Satisfaction After the First Baby Arrives." *Journal of Family Psychology,* 14, no. 1 (2000): 59–70. pdfs.semanticscholar.org/0fce/799e726ea33fd80a3859fde3e4eb7a40aec0.pdf?_ga=2.190745963.130843 7689.1593576249-1972260653.1592859511.

Tatkin, Stan. *Wired for Dating: How Understanding Neurobiology and Attachment Style Can Help You Find Your Ideal Mate.* Oakland, CA: New Harbinger, 2016.

———. *Wired for Love: How Understanding Your Partner's Brain and Attachment Style Can Help You Defuse Conflict and Build a Secure Relationship.* Oakland, CA: New Harbinger, 2012.

U.S. Census Bureau. "PINC-05. Work Experience—People 15 Years Old and Over, by Total Money Earnings, Age, Race, Hispanic Origin, Sex, and Disability Status." www.census.gov/data/tables/time-series/demo/income-poverty/cps-pinc/pinc-05.html.

Real change *is* possible

For more than forty-five years, New Harbinger has published proven-effective self-help books and pioneering workbooks to help readers of all ages and backgrounds improve mental health and well-being, and achieve lasting personal growth. In addition, our spirituality books offer profound guidance for deepening awareness and cultivating healing, self-discovery, and fulfillment.

Founded by psychologist Matthew McKay and Patrick Fanning, New Harbinger is proud to be an independent, employee-owned company. Our books reflect our core values of integrity, innovation, commitment, sustainability, compassion, and trust. Written by leaders in the field and recommended by therapists worldwide, New Harbinger books are practical, accessible, and provide real tools for real change.

 newharbingerpublications

Kara Hoppe, MA, MFT, is a psychotherapist, teacher, feminist, and mother. She has spent more than a decade as an inclusive therapist working with individuals and couples toward healing and growing; and toward becoming grounded, integrated people with better access to their own instincts, wisdom, and creativity. Hoppe currently lives in Pioneertown, CA; and sees clients in private practice via telehealth. You can learn more about her at www.karahoppe.com.

Stan Tatkin, PsyD, MFT, is a clinician, teacher, and developer of the Psychobiological Approach to Couple Therapy (PACT). He has a clinical practice in Calabasas, CA; where he has specialized for the last twenty years in working with couples and individuals who wish to be in relationships. He and his wife, Tracey Boldemann-Tatkin, developed the PACT Institute for the purpose of training other psychotherapists to use this method in their clinical work.

Foreword writer **Terry Real** is an internationally recognized family therapist, speaker, and author of *The New Rules of Marriage*.

MORE BOOKS from
NEW HARBINGER PUBLICATIONS

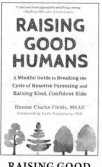
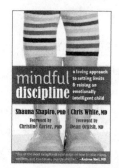
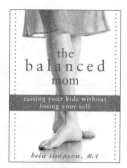
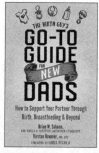
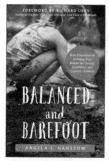
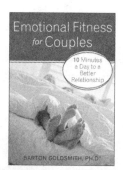